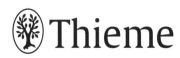

Digital Breast Tomosynthesis

Technique and Cases

Joerg Barkhausen, MD

Professor of Radiology
Department of Radiology and Nuclear Medicine
University of Lübeck
Lübeck, Germany

Achim Rody, MD

Professor of Obstetrics and Gynecology
Department of Obstetrics and Gynecology
University of Lübeck
Lübeck, Germany

Fritz K. W. Schaefer, MD

Professor of Radiology
Division of Breast Imaging and Interventions
Schleswig-Holstein University Hospital
Kiel Campus
Kiel, Germany

486 illustrations

Thieme
Stuttgart · New York · Delhi · Rio de Janeiro

Library of Congress Cataloging-in-Publication Data is available from the publisher.
This book is an authorized translation of the German edition published and copyrighted 2015 by Georg Thieme Verlag, Stuttgart. Title of the German edition: Digitale Tomosynthese der Brust

Translator: Terry C. Telger, Fort Worth, TX, USA
Illustrator: Karin Baum, Paphos, Cyprus

Important note: Medicine is an ever-changing science undergoing continual development. Research and clinical experience are continually expanding our knowledge, in particular our knowledge of proper treatment and drug therapy. Insofar as this book mentions any dosage or application, readers may rest assured that the authors, editors, and publishers have made every effort to ensure that such references are in accordance **with the state of knowledge at the time of production of the book.**

Nevertheless, this does not involve, imply, or express any guarantee or responsibility on the part of the publishers in respect to any dosage instructions and forms of applications stated in the book. **Every user is requested to examine carefully** the manufacturers' leaflets accompanying each drug and to check, if necessary in consultation with a physician or specialist, whether the dosage schedules mentioned therein or the contraindications stated by the manufacturers differ from the statements made in the present book. Such examination is particularly important with drugs that are either rarely used or have been newly released on the market. Every dosage schedule or every form of application used is entirely at the user's own risk and responsibility. The authors and publishers request every user to report to the publishers any discrepancies or inaccuracies noticed. If errors in this work are found after publication, errata will be posted at www.thieme.com on the product description page.

Some of the product names, patents, and registered designs referred to in this book are in fact registered trademarks or proprietary names even though specific reference to this fact is not always made in the text. Therefore, the appearance of a name without designation as proprietary is not to be construed as a representation by the publisher that it is in the public domain.

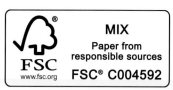

© 2016 Georg Thieme Verlag KG

Thieme Publishers Stuttgart
Rüdigerstrasse 14, 70469 Stuttgart, Germany
+49 [0]711 8931 421, customerservice@thieme.de

Thieme Publishers New York
333 Seventh Avenue, New York, NY 10001, USA
+1-800-782-3488, customerservice@thieme.com

Thieme Publishers Delhi
A-12, Second Floor, Sector-2, Noida-201301
Uttar Pradesh, India
+91 120 45 566 00, customerservice@thieme.in

Thieme Publishers Rio, Thieme Publicações Ltda.
Edifício Rodolpho de Paoli, 25º andar
Av. Nilo Peçanha, 50 – Sala 2508
Rio de Janeiro 20020-906 Brasil
+55 21 3172 2297 / +55 21 3172 1896

Cover design: Thieme Publishing Group
Typesetting by Druckhaus Götz GmbH, Ludwigsburg, Germany

Printed in Germany by Aprinta, Wemding

ISBN 978-3-13-203161-6   5 4 3 2 1

Also available as an e-book:
eISBN 978-3-13-203171-5

Contents

List of Videos

Foreword

Thirty years ago in 1985, after completing a radiology residency and fellowship, I was afforded an opportunity to develop the first patient-oriented breast imaging center in Pittsburgh, Pennsylvania, USA. One of my new colleagues, a general radiologist who had interpreted mammograms for many years, often articulated her yearning for "slices" to see better into the dense breast parenchyma within the routine screening projections. This was the era of renal tomography, an important component of the intravenous urogram (IVU) that antedated computed tomography (CT), precontrast for stones and postcontrast for parenchymal abnormalities, years before tomographic techniques applied to X-ray mammography were advanced sufficiently for clinical use in breast imaging.

What was mammography like then? In many radiology departments, the method of choice was xeromammography, a radiographic procedure performed with balloon compression, where the breast's image was recorded on thick paper. As women became aware of the benefits of breast cancer screening, the demand for mammography grew, and these light-blue xeromammograms were replaced by single-emulsion film, which required lower X-ray doses and was more suited to higher volumes. The xeromammography machines were sent to emergency departments, which used the low-contrast examinations for locating glass shards or splinters in soft tissues. The single-emulsion film had high spatial resolution with variable levels of contrast; this was enhanced by the use of grids, which increased the dose but reduced scatter, improving the signal-to-noise ratio. These films were interpreted on rotators with high luminance, or viewboxes, freestanding or wall mounted.

Gradually, the conversion from film to digital recording systems for cross-sectional imaging, and then all radiographic studies, forced the development of digital mammography, which had higher contrast resolution than film but lower spatial resolution, slowing adoption of digital mammography by breast imagers. The accuracy of film compared with digital mammography was studied in the American College of Radiology Imaging Network (ACRIN) DMIST study of nearly 50,000 women in North America, comparing film-screening mammography to digital mammography. The study concluded that digital mammography is more accurate than film in women under the age of 50 years, women with radiographically dense breasts, and pre- or perimenopausal women.[1]

The technologic advances underscored the need for further refinements and work continued on tomosynthesis, which now provided the thin projections my colleague had asked for many years earlier to help her decide between a summation density and a mass when explaining a finding on conventional two-dimensional mammography. As technical advances have continued, in the same time frame as publication of this clinically useful book three major manufacturers of tomosynthesis equipment have satisfied the rigorous regulatory requirements of image quality and dose and received approval of the United States Food and Drug Administration (FDA). The differences among the three different tomosynthesis systems are covered in this text, and, as the authors state, growing numbers of breast imagers have quickly and enthusiastically adopted this technology for both screening and diagnostic applications.

For new users of tomosynthesis, as well as those intending to integrate it into their breast-imaging workflow, this textbook offers the required knowledge in several chapters that detail the physics of tomosynthesis, discuss considerations of image quality and the reduction of screening recall rates, and look into concerns of dose, artifacts, interpretation time, cost effectiveness, and image archiving. With an emphasis on the technical progress that is being pursued actively, the authors provide a summary of the literature that has appeared on both sides of the Atlantic, adding the recently reported results of a large retrospective multicenter study of nearly 455,000 women that confirmed a decrease in screening recall rates and an increase in cancer detection[2]. These chapters are illustrated with beautiful images, but the book's uniqueness lies in its presentation, with videoclips, of 45 tomosynthesis teaching cases, some of which are multimodality; these will equip readers with experience that is as close as possible to personal clinical experience.

Professors Barkhausen, Rody, and Schaefer should be congratulated on providing solid information to the breast health care team that will enable informed decisions about whether or not tomosynthesis should have a place among the modalities offered for screening and diagnosis of breast cancer in their facility's practice. The benefits and weaknesses of the systems available for clinical use are summarized. As technical refinements continue, and data on sensitivity and specificity validate tomosynthesis, this well-written book will be a valuable resource. It is a pleasure to read and, especially, to lose oneself voyaging through the many beautifully prepared teaching cases that provide a virtual clinical experience.

Ellen B. Mendelson, MD, FACR, FSBI
Lee F. Rogers
Professor of Medical Education in Radiology
Professor of Radiology
Feinberg School of Medicine
Northwestern University
Chicago, Illinois, USA

[1] Pisano ED, Gatsonis CA, Hendrick RE et al. Diagnostic performance of digital versus film mammography for breast-cancer screening. N Engl J Med 2005;353 (17):1773–83
[2] Friedewald SM, Rafferty EA, Rose SL et al. Breast Cancer screening using tomosythesis in combination with digital mammography. JAMA 2014;311 (24):2499-2507

Preface

Digital breast tomosynthesis has been available for routine clinical use for 5 years now, and there is still no textbook devoted to this innovative technology. We want to remedy that!

This book examines the results of existing clinical studies on digital breast tomosynthesis and, based on those findings, offers sound recommendations for its routine clinical use. The second part of the book presents 45 illustrative case reports, enabling our readers to explore the practical aspects of tomosynthesis, as well as deepening and testing their clinical knowledge. We felt it was important to present high-quality images from all available modalities in breast imaging, so that the strengths and limitations of the various techniques could be compared and discussed.

Successful breast imaging relies on interdisciplinary teamwork between radiologists and gynecologists, who review their findings in tumor board meetings with pathologists, oncologists, and radiation oncologists. We followed this interdisciplinary approach in our selection of authors and editors: Diagnosticians and clinicians practiced in the everyday use of tomosynthesis have pooled their many years of experience, especially in compiling the illustrative case reports.

This book is intended for physicians in continuing education and for colleagues who are experienced in breast diagnosis and want to familiarize themselves with these new techniques in breast imaging. May our readers find the book both instructive and enjoyable!

Joerg Barkhausen
Achim Rody
Fritz Schaefer

Contributors

Joerg Barkhausen, MD
Professor of Radiology
Department of Radiology and Nuclear Medicine
University of Lübeck
Lübeck, Germany

Kristin Baumann, MD
Department of Obstetrics and Gynecology
University of Lübeck
Lübeck, Germany

Dorothea Fischer, MD
Associate Professor of Obstetrics and Gynecology
Department of Obstetrics and Gynecology
University of Lübeck
Lübeck, Germany

Isabell Grande-Nagel, MD
Department of Radiology and Nuclear Medicine
University of Lübeck
Lübeck, Germany

Smaragda Kapsimalakou, MD
Department of Radiology and Nuclear Medicine
University of Lübeck
Lübeck, Germany

Thomas Mertelmeier, PhD
Siemens AG Healthcare Sector
Clinical Products Division, X-Ray Products
H CP XP R&D TEC
Erlangen, Germany

Christoph Mundhenke, MD
Professor of Obstetrics and Gynecology
Department of Obstetrics and Gynecology
Schleswig-Holstein University Hospital
Kiel Campus
Kiel, Germany

Berndt Michael Order, MD
Division of Breast Imaging and Interventions
Schleswig-Holstein University Hospital
Kiel Campus
Kiel, Germany

Achim Rody, MD
Professor of Obstetrics and Gynecology
Department of Obstetrics and Gynecology
University of Lübeck
Lübeck, Germany

Fritz K. W. Schaefer, MD
Professor of Radiology
Division of Breast Imaging and Interventions
Schleswig-Holstein University Hospital
Kiel Campus
Kiel, Germany

Florian Vogt, MD
Associate Professor of Radiology
Department of Radiology and Nuclear Medicine
University of Lübeck
Lübeck, Germany

Abbreviations

2D	two dimensional
3D	three dimensional
AAPM	American Association of Physicists in Medicine
ACR	American College of Radiology (score for radiographic breast density)
AGD	average glandular dose
ART	algebraic reconstruction technique
a-Si	amorphous silicon
AUC	area under the ROC curve
BCS	breast-conserving surgery
BI-RADS	Breast Imaging Reporting and Data System (scores level of cancer suspicion)
CAD	computer-aided detection
CC	craniocaudal
CE	Communauté Européenne (European Community)
CT	computed tomography
DBT	digital breast tomosynthesis
DCIS	ductal carcinoma in situ
DgN	normalized glandular dose
DQE	detective quantum efficiency
EUREF	European Reference Organization for Quality Assured Breast Screening and Diagnostic Services
FBP	filtered back projection
FFDM	full-field digital mammography
Gx, Px	number of pregnancies (G, gravida) and number of deliveries (P, para)
Gy	gray
HRT	hormone replacement therapy
HU	Hounsfield unit
IEC	International Electrotechnical Commission
kVp	peak kilovoltage
LIN	lobular intraepithelial neoplasia
mAs	milliampere–second
MB	megabyte
mGy	milligray
ML	mediolateral
MLO	mediolateral oblique
MR	magnetic resonance
MRI	magnetic resonance imaging
NST	of no special type
ROC	receiver operating characteristic (curve)
SART	simultaneous algebraic reconstruction technique
SD	standard deviation
SIRT	simultaneous iterative reconstruction technique
TFT	thin-film transistor
VAB	vacuum-assisted biopsy
W/Al	tungsten/aluminum
W/Rh	tungsten/rhodium

Glossary

Aliasing Streak artifacts due to a limited number of projections

Artifact Spurious signal

Autologous Belonging to the same individual

Benign Noncancerous

Fulcrum Point around which the X-ray source rotates in the focal plane

Glandularity Proportion of glandular tissue relative to all tissue

Kerma Kinetic energy released per unit mass. Ratio of the kinetic energy transmitted to first-generation secondary particles divided by the irradiated mass

Air kerma Measurement of the kerma, using air as a reference medium

Malignant Cancerous

Moiré effect Special case of the aliasing effect caused by undersampling

Mortality Death rate

Incidence Number of new cases of a given disease in one year

Pixel Smallest picture element displayed in a digitized raster image

Recall Call-back of a patient for additional testing

Shepp–Logan filter Combination of a ramp filter and spectral filter in computed tomography

Voxel Volume element, an image point within the volume of a scan

Chapter 1

Introduction

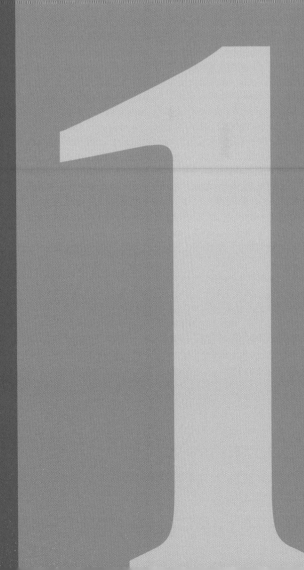

1 Introduction

Joerg Barkhausen and Achim Rody

In 2012, 1.7 million women worldwide were diagnosed with breast cancer and there were 6.3 million women alive who had been diagnosed with breast cancer in the previous 5 years. Today, breast cancer is the most common cause of cancer death among women (522,000 deaths in 2012) and the most frequently diagnosed cancer among women worldwide.[1] Over the last 5 years, the incidence of breast cancer has increased by 14%. Possible reasons for this effect, besides biological factors, are mammographic screening, early detection, and significant advances in diagnostic imaging. Digital mammography, high-resolution breast ultrasonography, image-guided interventional procedures, and magnetic resonance mammography are among the standard techniques now available as a complementary protocol for curative diagnosis and screening. These technologies have advanced greatly in the past decade and are now applied on a population-wide scale, with quality assurance, for indications that are clearly specified in official guidelines.

However, currently established routine techniques and algorithms cannot always positively distinguish between benign and malignant lesions. This is illustrated by the interval cancers that develop after screening and by the high rate of negative breast biopsies, which exceeds 50% in some settings. This points to a need for further optimization of existing modalities, as well as a need to develop entirely new imaging techniques. More than 15 years after it was first described, digital breast tomosynthesis (DBT) has now entered routine clinical use.

New techniques always pose a challenge. On the one hand, they invite us to scrutinize more traditional studies. On the other, they compel us to define the patients, settings, and indications for which the new technique would be medically appropriate and economically feasible. Many of these questions on the routine clinical use of tomosynthesis cannot yet be definitively answered. This book explains the technique of tomosynthesis, describes the principal results of available clinical studies, and explores the next evolutionary steps in this technology. The explanatory chapters are followed by numerous case reports in Chapter 5, most with histologic confirmation, that will illustrate both the capabilities and limitations of breast tomosynthesis.

The key question, of course, is whether DBT is basically an adjunctive technique or whether it can replace digital mammography in the near future. A major goal in screening is to reduce recall rates and false-positive results. The detection rates of DBT need clarification for different histologic or even molecular subtypes in curative mammography. Its impact on surgical treatment planning must also be tested, especially with regard to the detection of multicentric disease. Autologous and alloplastic breast reconstructions are a particular challenge in terms of follow-up. Finally, it is essential to determine the reliability of tomosynthesis in the detection of recurrent disease.

It will definitely take time to answer all of these questions. One thing is certain, however: DBT is a fascinating technology that will continue to draw great clinical and scientific interest in the years ahead.

1.1 References

[1] Ferlay J, Soerjomataram I, Ervik M, et al. GLOBOCAN 2012 v1.0, Estimated Cancer Incidence, Mortality, and Prevalence Worldwide in 2012: IARC CancerBase No. 11 [Internet]. Lyon: International Agency for Research on Cancer; 2013. Available at: http://globocan.iarc.fr. Accessed May 6, 2015

Chapter 2

The Physics of Tomosynthesis

2 The Physics of Tomosynthesis

Thomas Mertelmeier

2.1 Introduction

A few years after the discovery of X-rays by Wilhelm C. Röntgen, researchers began to consider how this radiation might be used not only to create projection radiographs but also to supply three-dimensional (3D) information on the object of interest. Many years passed, however, before this idea became a technical reality. In the first 3D technique, the X-ray source was moved relative to the object, to generate a summation image on the receptor (film) of the X-rays attenuated by the object. In this technique, known as tomography or conventional tomography (Greek *tomos* = "slice" or "section"), the radiation source moves around a pivot point (fulcrum) in the focal plane. This motion keeps the plane of interest in sharp focus, while blurring out tissues above and below that level.

Ziedses des Plantes made the first practical use of linear-motion tomography for imaging the skull.[1] The source and detector moved around the fulcrum in a linear fashion. As a result, Ziedses des Plantes is often recognized as the founder of tomography, even though there were many other variants of the technique.[2,3]

A major disadvantage of conventional tomography was the high radiation dose required, since only one plane was in focus, as determined by the acquisition geometry. Each additional image slice required a different acquisition geometry to define the new plane of interest. This situation did not change until the advent of digital image receptors (flat-panel detectors), which permitted a rapid and distortion-free data readout. The desired image slice could then be reconstructed retrospectively by computer, from the individual stored projection images. This technology provides an obvious reduction in dose, since any desired image plane can be imaged sharply with just one movement of the acquisition system. This technique, in which the X-ray source occupies various imaging positions relative to the object, is called *digital tomosynthesis* or simply *tomosynthesis*. Sectional images are reconstructed from a set of individual projection images that are acquired at different angles. This allows the user to "look around" structures within the object to obtain 3D information in the form of individual image slices.

The main advantage of tomosynthesis is its ability to select discrete tissue planes. This principle is illustrated in **Fig. 2.1**, which shows images reconstructed from a breast data set. The image plane in **Fig. 2.1a** is located 23 mm above the breast support plate ($z = 23$ mm). It clearly demonstrates a round lesion with smooth margins. The clustered microcalcifications above the lesion are only faintly visible. They are clearly depicted in **Fig. 2.1b**, however, where the image plane is 27 mm above the support plate ($z = 27$ mm), whereas the round lesion itself is poorly visualized. This ability to select individual tissue planes could increase both the detection rate and the level of diagnostic confidence. Niklason et al described one of the first applications for breast imaging as early as 1997.[4]

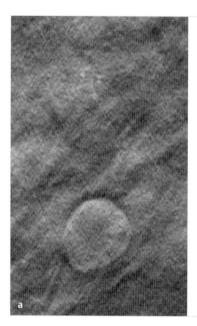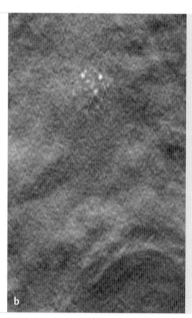

Fig. 2.1 Magnified views (18 × 29 mm) of two tomosynthesis slices in the breast. (Raw data were provided courtesy of Dr. Ingvar Andersson, Malmö University Hospital, Sweden, and Siemens AG Healthcare Sector.) **(a)** Image slice at level $z = 23$ mm. The round lesion is in focus. **(b)** Image slice at level $z = 27$ mm. The clustered microcalcifications are in focus.

2.2 Data Acquisition and Scanning

Modified X-ray systems are most commonly used for to-mosynthesis. Breast tomosynthesis may employ digital mammographic systems in which the X-ray source can be moved, occupying various positions relative to the im-aged object (breast).

Tomosynthesis systems can operate in one of two modes. In the sweep mode, the X-ray tube moves contin-uously and is pulsed at the frame rate of the detector. In the "step-and-shoot" mode, the tube moves to the next position betweeen two aquisitions and transmits the X-ray pulse while the tube is stationary. The tube may move in an arc around a point within the object, or at least close to the object, or it may move along a linear path. During scan acquisition, the detector may be stationary (**Fig. 2.2**) or may move simultaneously with the tube. In the case of a moving detector, the system may have an isocentric C-arm geometry, in which the detector and source both rotate around a common point, or it may have a partial isocentric geometry. In this type of system, the tube and detector move in a synchronous way, but the detector is not rigidly connected to the tube. For ex-ample, it may move on a linear path in the receptor plane.[5] In most imaging systems, the breast is positioned close to the detector, so there is little or no synchronous movement of the detector (**Fig. 2.2**).

Because each individual projection contributes to form-ing an image point within the scanned volume (volume element, voxel) during image reconstruction, a tomosyn-thesis data set can be acquired at approximately the same dose as a two-dimensional (2D) projection radiograph (see Chapter 2.5). The total exposure is distributed over the individual projections, however, so the detector must be able to supply a low-noise signal even at low dose lev-els. This means that the detector must have high detec-tive quantum efficiency (DQE), even at a very low dose (see Chapter 2.5). Moreover, the detector must have a fast readout and high frame rate, to minimize the scan time and shorten the necessary breast-compression time.[6] Both detector requirements pose a significant challenge, given the spatial and contrast resolution required for breast imaging. The scan time can be shortened by "bin-ning" the pixels during detector readout. The associated loss of resolution and possible increase in the signal-to-noise ratio depend on the technical details of the system in use.

Breast tomosynthesis systems currently on the market (see example in **Fig. 2.3**) employ direct-conversion detec-tors based on amorphous selenium with thin-film tran-sistor (TFT) arrays made of amorphous silicon (a-Si-TFT). There is also a system with a scintillator and photodiodes made of amorphous silicon with a-Si-TFT readout arrays, as well as a prototype scanner equipped with silicon di-rect-conversion line detectors.

The X-ray spectrum used for tomosynthesis is either the same as, or similar to, that used in digital mammogra-phy, and the tube voltage depends on the thickness of the compressed breast. The X-ray energy, or tube voltage, may be increased slightly to keep the dose as low as pos-sible. Another option is to use more filtering, which in-creases the mean quantum energy. Tungsten/rhodium (W/Rh) is a typical anode/filter combination. Tungsten/ aluminum (W/Al) can also be used.

Vertical image resolution and depth of focus depend mainly on the acquisition geometry, i.e., the tomosynthe-sis angle (**Fig. 2.4**). The tomosynthesis angle is defined as the angular range over which the X-ray tube is moved rel-ative to the pivot point. The greater the tomosynthesis angle, the better the depth resolution and the smaller the effective slice thickness. This results in less image blurring from adjacent tissues due to out-of-plane artifacts. A large tomosynthesis angle can also improve contrast res-olution at low spatial frequencies (i.e., for relatively large objects) because the greater angular range can supply more information, especially at small spatial frequencies (see Chapter 2.3).[7,8] It should be added, however, that a stationary detector that does not move simultaneously with the tube will reduce the accessible scan volume, ow-ing to the oblique incidence of the X-ray beams.

It is not possible to state an "optimum" angular range, because depth resolution is not the only parameter af-fected by the tomosynthesis angle. For example, a large tomosynthesis angle prolongs the scan time for a given angular velocity of the X-ray tube, increasing the risk of motion artifacts. Current scanners have tomosynthesis

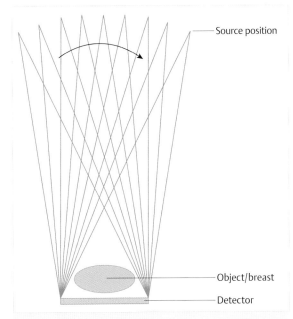

Fig. 2.2 Tomosynthesis acquisition geometry with a stationary detector and nine source positions or projections.

Source position

Object/breast

Detector

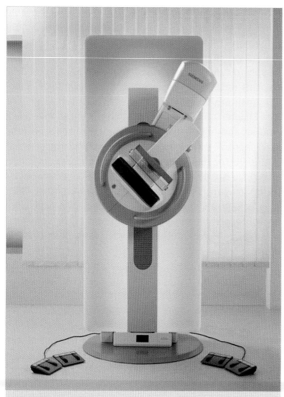

Fig. 2.3 Breast tomosynthesis scanner, shown in the medio-lateral-oblique position.

angles between 11 and 60°, all of which yield good results. To date, however, there have been no systematic clinical studies on how the tomosynthesis angle affects the detection of clinically relevant structures (spiculated lesions, microcalcifications) in the breast.

In addition to the limited angular range, the limited number of projections (sparse sampling) presents a challenge for 3D scanners. In the imaging of high-contrast objects, undersampling leads to Moiré effects (aliasing), which appear as streak artifacts similar to those seen in computed tomography (CT). The principle is the same in tomosynthesis, where the angular increment between exposures should not exceed several degrees, in order to prevent streak artifacts. In practice, the maximum number of projections is determined by the minimum dose at the detector per exposure to yield a total dose comparable to that of a conventional mammogram. The scan time, which translates to breast-compression time for the patient, depends on the number of projections for a given detector frame rate. Current tomosynthesis scanners, including prototypes, usually acquire between 7 and 30 projections in one examination.

Thus, the following quantities depend on acquisition geometry, scan parameters, and system hardware components:

- Resolution.
- Noise.
- Artifact level.
- Dose.
- Accessible volume.
- Examination time.

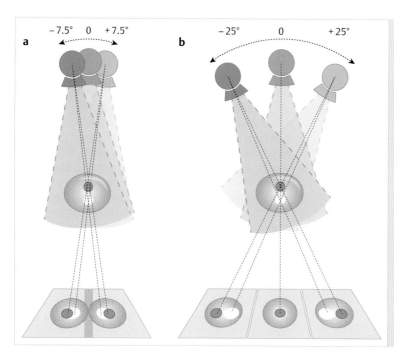

Fig. 2.4 Effect of the tomosynthesis angle on depth resolution. **(a)** A small tomosynthesis angle gives poorer separation of adjacent object points in the vertical direction. **(b)** A large tomosynthesis angle provides better separation of adjacent points in the vertical direction.

All these quantities require optimization of the entire system. A survey published by Sechopoulos in 2013[9,10] provides an up-to-date technical review of breast tomosynthesis that covers all aspects of this topic—from acquisition geometry and detector technology, to the X-ray spectrum, dose, and image reconstruction. The article also surveys systems in current use.

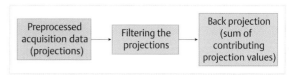

Fig. 2.5 Flowchart for analytical reconstruction by the filtered back-projection method.

2.3 Image Reconstruction

In tomosynthesis image reconstruction, the spatial distribution of the n-dimensional attenuation coefficient of the object is computed from $(n-1)$-dimensional projection images of the n-dimensional object acquired at different angles. Since the acquisition of tomosynthesis data is based on 2D projection images, the 3D attenuation coefficient is computed. Owing to the limited angular range of data acquisition (limited-angle tomography), this problem cannot be solved exactly, but its solution can be closely approximated using mathematical methods. Also, there is no objective, quantitative grayscale unit for the reconstructed slices that is comparable to the Hounsfield unit (HU) used in CT.

Moreover, the limited tomosynthesis angle makes it impossible to achieve isotropic resolution. Resolution is lower in the direction of the central ray, hereafter called the vertical or z-axis, than along the x- and y-axes, because projections characterized by an angle larger than the tomosynthesis angle, which carry the additional information necessary for isotropic depth resolution, are not measured. As a result, only image slices that are perpendicular to the vertical axis are reconstructed in tomosynthesis. In systems with a stationary detector, these slices are parallel to the detector plane.

In principle, two broad classes of method are available for tomosynthesis reconstruction:
- Analytical reconstruction.
- Iterative reconstruction.

2.3.1 Analytical Reconstruction

Analytical algorithms for tomosynthesis reconstruction are based on standard algorithms used in CT. Analytical methods employ specially designed reconstruction filters to compensate for scanning over a limited angular range and minimize artifacts. Various algorithms for tomosynthesis reconstruction have been described in the literature.[5,11,12] The methods are called "analytical" because the solution is formulated analytically using an inverse Radon transformation. This solution is then fed into a computer and calculated by numerical methods. The basic technique for this type of reconstruction is described next (**Fig. 2.5**).[13]

First, the projection images necessary for slice reconstruction are determined from the 2D acquisition data, by taking the logarithm and by normalization with the non-attenuated intensity. According to Beer's attenuation law, the projections necessary for the inverse Radon transform are represented by the line integrals through the object for rays that connect the X-ray focus to a point on the detector. These 2D projections are transformed with suitable reconstruction filters, to obtain filtered projection values. For better computer efficiency, this filtering is usually done by Fourier transformation in frequency space. The filtered projections are then back projected into the object volume (filtered back projection, FBP).

This means that for a given voxel in the object volume, all projection values whose rays run precisely through that voxel, and thus contribute to the image, are summed and then averaged. The filter consists of a ramp filter like that used in CT. It has the property of inverting the ideal 2D CT problem, i.e., compensating for blurring caused by the angular sampling scheme, based on the acquisition geometry. However, because the ramp filter amplifies the high spatial frequencies, it also increases image noise. These high spatial frequencies must therefore be suppressed with a "spectral filter." CT employs a combination of both filter types (ramp filter and spectral filter) called the Shepp–Logan filter.[13]

Because the tomosynthesis problem does not have an exact mathematical solution, different FBP techniques use different filter designs, leading to differences in image appearance and artifact suppression.[14,15,16,17] **Fig. 2.6** illustrates how different filter designs can affect the appearance of an image. **Fig. 2.6a** shows a tomosynthesis slice reconstructed with an edge-enhancing filter, generating an image that resembles a CT scan. **Fig. 2.6b** shows the same slice from the same data set, reconstructed with a different filter. By accentuating the glandular breast tissue, this image looks more like a mammogram.

2.3.2 Iterative Reconstruction

Unlike analytical reconstruction, iterative techniques solve the inverse problem by first formulating the system equation for the relationship between the object and projection data, as an algebraic equation in the form of a large system of equations, and then solving it numerically. Because the system of equations is extremely large, it can only be solved with iterative techniques. As the iterations are carried out, the projection values computed from the object of interest are compared with the measured projection values in each iterative step. Based on the

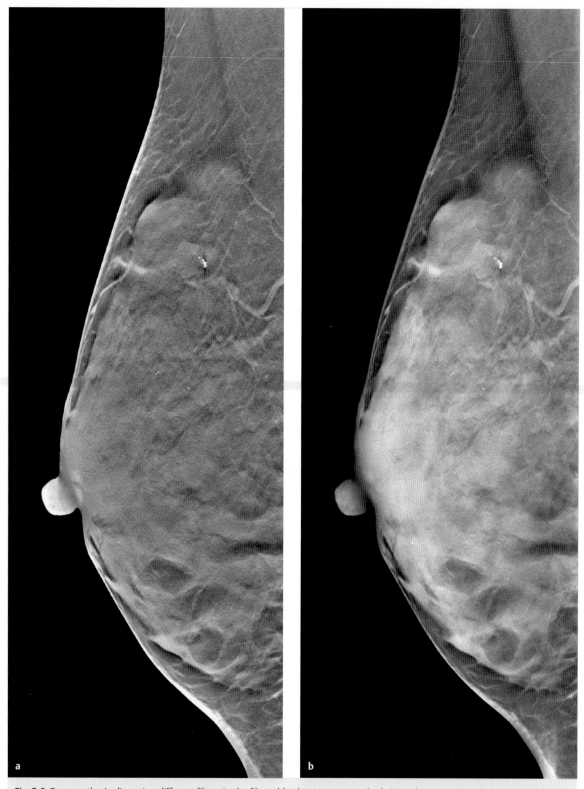

Fig. 2.6 Tomosynthesis slice using different filters in the filtered back-projection method. (Raw data were provided courtesy of Dr. Nachiko Uchiyama, National Cancer Center, Tokyo, Japan, and Siemens AG Healthcare Sector.) **(a)** Edge-enhanced image. **(b)** Accentuation of glandular breast tissue.

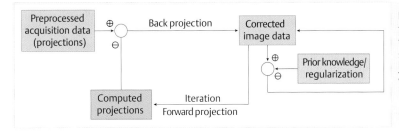

Fig. 2.7 Flowchart for iterative reconstruction. Based on an initial estimated value for the image data, the final image is reconstructed iteratively by using forward projection, prior knowledge, and comparison with the acquisition data.

discrepancy, the object distribution is improved in a step-by-step fashion, until the solution fulfills a certain optimality criterion (**Fig. 2.7**). This can be done by various iterative methods, such as the algebraic reconstruction technique (ART), simultaneous ART (SART),[18] or simultaneous iterative reconstruction technique (SIRT). By basing the formulation of the problem on the Poisson statistics for X-ray quanta, a statistical iterative method can be supplied, using a "maximum-likelihood" reconstruction algorithm.[19] Additionally, constraints and prior knowledge may be available during the solution process. This yields a more stable solution with low image noise (maximum a posteriori methods or penalized maximum-likelihood algorithms).

All these iterative techniques differ in their update strategies, i.e., how the solution is successively improved in each iterative step, what constraints are assumed, available prior knowledge, and the numerical solution techniques.

2.3.3 Combined Reconstruction Methods

Besides these main classes of analytical and iterative reconstructions, there are a number of modified algorithms that combine analytical methods with iterative algebraic techniques. The goal of these methods is to keep blurring and other artifacts to an absolute minimum. Examples of methods used in breast tomosynthesis are iterative deblurring[20,21] and nonlinear back projection.[22,23]

2.3.4 Visualization

Regardless of the type of reconstruction used, tomosynthesis always generates a nonisotropic volume data set, in which vertical resolution is much poorer than in planes perpendicular to the optical axis. Because most artifacts also occur in the vertical direction, image slices parallel to the detector are best for visualization. Thus, viewing multiple sequential slices in the "stack mode" is preferred. True volume rendering is only possible over a very limited angular range that is roughly equal to the tomosynthesis angle.

Compared with digital mammography, the size of an image data set in tomosynthesis poses a definite challenge in both the reconstruction and viewing of images. If

the detector has a 2800×3600 pixel matrix at 16 bits per pixel, this gives 20 megabytes (MB) of raw data per projection. A raw data set with N_p projections would require a storage capacity of $N_p \times 20$ MB. For 15 projections, this would be 300 MB.

Typically, the images are reconstructed with a slice separation of 1 mm, and the reconstructed pixel size in the image plane should never be larger than one detector pixel. The average size of an image slice is slightly smaller than that of one projection, because the average breast does not cover the whole detector. Assuming, for example, that a reconstructed tomosynthesis slice consists of 2000×3000 pixels, 12 MB (at 16 bits per pixel) are obtained for the data content of one slice. An average compressed breast thickness of 50 mm would result in 50 slices containing 600 MB of data. In this example, then, a data set consisting of raw projections plus reconstructed slices would be 900 MB in size. A complete examination in four planes (left and right, craniocaudal, lateral oblique) would require 3600 MB of storage. The exact figure will vary depending on specific technical details (detector size, pixel size, number of projections, slice interval).

2.4 Artifacts

Because the object is not sampled completely in tomosynthesis, owing to the limited angular range, the inverse problem cannot be solved exactly. This undersampling leads to artifacts that result mainly from the fact that the point spread function deviates from spherical symmetry. As a result, point objects will be spread along the vertical z-axis and extend over multiple planes. Since the individual projections are also separated from one another by a finite angular increment (usually a few degrees), these artifacts are not distributed uniformly but reflect the individual projections. They are called "out-of-plane artifacts" because they cause unwanted visualization of structures outside the plane of interest.

Fig. 2.8a shows a calcification in the focal plane. The calcification is still visible several slices above or below the image plane, appearing as out-of-plane artifacts with a typical replicated structure (**Fig. 2.8b**). The intensity of these artifacts depends on the size and contrast of the object. The larger the structure, the more the artifact is spread out along the z-axis, affecting more slices adjacent

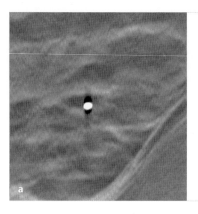
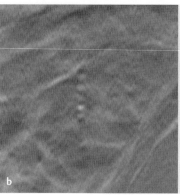

Fig. 2.8 Magnified views (30 × 30 mm) of an approximately 1.5-mm calcification in two tomosynthesis slices. (Raw data were provided courtesy of Dr. Jay Baker, Duke University Medical Center, Durham, NC, and Siemens AG Healthcare Sector.) **(a)** The calcification is in sharp focus. Dark-rim artifacts, aligned in the scan direction, are visible at the edge of the calcification. **(b)** Out-of-plane artifacts from the calcification are faintly visible in an adjacent slice 8 mm from the previous plane.

to the in-focus plane. The higher the contrast, the greater the intensity of the artifacts.

Missing data also produce another kind of artifact that results from the reconstruction filters. The frequency domain can be divided into a scanned region and an unscanned region. At the boundary between the two regions, filtering may produce overshoot or undershoot artifacts that appear as dark rims on a high-contrast object. The dark rims are lined up in the scan direction (**Fig. 2.8a**). Dark-rim artifacts are visible on a spiculated mass in **Fig. 2.9** and at the top and bottom of the round lesion in **Fig. 2.1a**.

In theory, the relatively low sampling density can lead to streak artifacts like those occurring in CT. However, these effects are usually minor in breast tomosynthesis, because they occur predominantly at high-contrast objects such as bone or metal. Since the breast consists of fat and glandular tissue, it is a low-contrast object with relatively homogeneous X-ray attenuation coefficients. Streak artifacts would be seen mainly in reformatted vertical slices, which are not displayed in tomosynthesis, owing to the poor vertical resolution.

While artifacts are unavoidable in tomosynthesis, there are situations in which they can aid image interpretation. As the reader is scrolling through a data set in stack mode, the presence of artifacts may accentuate relevant structures and make them easier to detect. The temporal contrast sensitivity of the human visual system is an important factor in this regard; it is maximal at frame rates from 1/s to 10/s, depending on luminance.[24] It should also be noted that an unsharp structure appearing in a sharp image always originates from an object outside the plane of focus and is not located in the slice of current interest. Thus, when viewing a single slice or scrolling through a stack of image slices, the reader should concentrate on sharply imaged structures and disregard blurred structures.

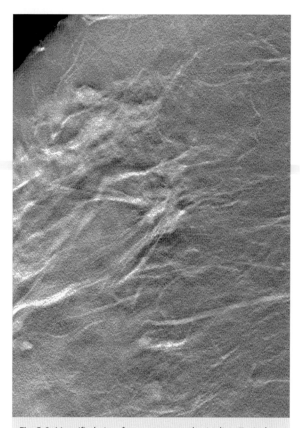

Fig. 2.9 Magnified view from a tomosynthesis slice. Typical dark-rim artifacts are visible at the upper and lower margins of the breast lesion. (Raw data were provided courtesy of Dr. Jay Baker, Duke University Medical Center, Durham, NC, and Siemens AG Healthcare Sector.)

2.5 Dose

The noise in a digital radiographic image is composed of quantum noise plus the noise from the readout electronics of the detector. Relative quantum noise is indirectly proportional to radiation dose, while the electronic noise is largely constant from one image to the next. In tomosynthesis, each individual projection is acquired at a much lower dose than in digital 2D mammography. This low dose significantly increases the relative quantum noise in each individual projection compared with a 2D mammogram, and the electronic noise of the detector accumulates with each additional projection.

One goal in tomosynthesis is to produce 3D information at approximately the same dose as that required for 2D mammography. This is only feasible if the noise in each individual projection image is determined almost entirely by quantum noise, with minimal electronic noise from detector readout. This is necessary to ensure that repeated detector readouts for the individual projections will not add too much cumulative electronic noise. When this condition is satisfied, the individual projections can be used to reconstruct an image slice that is comparable in noise level to a 2D digital mammogram. However, because electronic noise cannot be completely eliminated in practice, the tomosynthesis dose will always be slightly higher than the 2D mammogram dose, to achieve equal noise levels. This is why high-efficiency detectors with minimal readout noise are considered an essential prerequisite for tomosynthesis.

The average parenchymal dose in 2D projection mammography is usually estimated from the "average glandular dose" (AGD), which is determined on the basis of tabulated values[25,26]:

$$AGD = K \cdot g \cdot c \cdot s \tag{2.1}$$

In this equation, g transforms the incident dose at the breast surface, expressed in terms of the air kerma K, into the average glandular dose, with the correction factor c for breast glandularity. The factor s is an additional parameter taking into account the anode/filter combination. The air kerma can be measured or determined from the tube output (Gy/mAs) or current–time product (mAs). The factors g, c, and s have been determined by a Monte Carlo simulation of the absorbed dose in a breast model, for various beam qualities (half-value layers) and compressed breast thicknesses, and have been published in tables.[27]

A similar approach, also based on Monte Carlo simulations, has been presented by Wu et al and Boone.[28,29,30] In this method, the normalized glandular dose coefficients (DgN) are determined for various energies, breast thicknesses, and X-ray spectra and are used to convert the entrance ion dose to a glandular dose.

These approaches can be transferred from 2D imaging to tomosynthesis, although it must be considered that the projections enter the breast at nonperpendicular angles. Since the beams take different paths through the breast, they lead to different absorbed dose values than in 2D mammography.

Both methods based on Monte Carlo simulations for the spread of quanta in breast models have been applied to tomosynthesis,[31,32] and the results of both studies show good agreement. The methods take into account the special conditions of tomosynthesis, by using correction factors for parenchymal dose that depend on acquisition geometry and have been tabulated in the publications cited above. To summarize the results: For a given breast thickness and the same tube voltage (kVp) and total current–time product (mAs) as in 2D mammography, the radiation dose with current tomosynthesis acquisition geometries differs from 2D imaging by a factor of 0.9 to 1. In other words, calculating the average parenchymal dose just as in 2D mammography, yields an upper dose limit for breast tomosynthesis.

2.6 Overview of Existing Systems

Several breast tomosynthesis systems are currently available commercially and have come into clinical use, while other scanners are still in the prototype stage. All the systems differ in their acquisition geometries, detector technologies, and imaging processing and reconstruction.[9,10] Because breast tomosynthesis is a new technology with a vast innovative potential, it is reasonable to expect significant advances in the years ahead. **Table 2.1** reviews the technical specifications of scanners currently on the market.

2.7 Technical Quality Assurance

In Europe and many other parts of the world, a commercial product can be approved on the basis of Communauté Européenne (CE) certification, which documents its safety and effectiveness. At the present time, however, there are no uniform guidelines for technical quality assurance in tomosynthesis. In Germany, the *Quality Assurance Guideline* in the *X-Ray Ordinance* is applicable to tomosynthesis.[33] Additional quality-assurance measures can be found in the quality-control manuals supplied by the manufacturers.

In Europe, the European Reference Organization for Quality Assured Breast Screening and Diagnostic Services (EUREF) has been active in the field of quality assurance for breast tomosynthesis. An initial draft, still preliminary, was published in February 2013.[34] Another

Table 2.1 Main technical parameters of current tomosynthesis systems (as of July 2013), modified from Sechopoulos 2013[9,10]

Parameters	GE Healthcare	Hologic Dimensions	IMS Giotto	Philips Microdose	Siemens Mammomat Inspiration
Status	CE-certified	CE-certified	CE-certified	Prototype	CE-certified
Tomosynthesis angle	25°	15°	40°	11°	50°
Number of projections	9	15	13	21	25
Tube motion	Step & shoot	Continuous	Step & shoot	Continuous	Continuous
Scan time (s)	7	4	12	3–10	25
Detector size (cm²)	24 × 30	24 × 29	24 × 30	Multiple line detectors	24 × 30
Detector pixel (µm)	100	140	85	50	85
X-ray converter	CsI/a-Si	a-Se	a-Se	Si	a-Se
Radiation	Rh/Rh	W/Al	W/Rh	W/Al	W/Rh

Abbreviations: Al: aluminum, a-Se: amorphous selenium, a-Si: amorphous silicon, CE: Communauté Européenne, CsI: cesium iodide, Rh: rhodium, Si: silicon, W: tungsten.

international initiative is the work of Maintenance Team 31 of the International Electrotechnical Commission (IEC), relating to the standardization of quality assurance in mammography. In the academic community, the American Association of Physicists in Medicine (AAPM) has formed a Tomosynthesis Subcommittee that is working to place quality assurance on a scientific basis. For now we must await further developments, which will undoubtedly lead to the establishment of national and international standards in the next few years.

2.8 References

[1] Ziedses des Plantes BG. Een bijzondere methode voor het maken van Röntgenphoto's van schedel en wervelkolom. Ned Tijdschr Geneesk 1931; 75: 5218–5222

[2] Webb S. From the watching of shadows. The origins of radiological tomography. Bristol and New York: Adam Hilger; 1990

[3] Härer W, Lauritsch G, Mertelmeier T. Tomografie – Prinzip und Potenzial der Schichtbildverfahren. In: Schmidt T (editor). Handbuch Diagnostische Radiologie, Bd. 1, Strahlenphysik, Strahlenbiologie, Strahlenschutz. Berlin: Springer; 2001: 191–199

[4] Niklason LT, Christian BD, Niklason LE et al. Digital tomosynthesis in breast imaging. Radiology 1997; 205: 399–406

[5] Dobbins JT III, Godfrey DJ. Digital X-ray tomosynthesis: current state of the art and clinical potential. Phys Med Biol 2003; 48: R65 –R106

[6] Bissonnette M, Hansroul M, Masson E et al. Digital breast tomosynthesis using an amorphous selenium flat panel detector. Proc SPIE 2005; 5745: 529–540

[7] Zhao B, Zhou J, Hu Y-H et al. Experimental validation of a three-dimensional linear system model for breast tomosynthesis. Med Phys 2009; 36: 240–251

[8] Mertelmeier T, Ludwig J, Zhao B et al. Optimization of tomosynthesis acquisition parameters: angular range and number of projections. In: Krupinski E (editor). Lecture Notes in Computer Science 5116, Digital Mammography, 9th International Workshop, IWDM 2008. Berlin, Heidelberg: Springer; 2008: 220–227

[9] Sechopoulos I. A review of breast tomosynthesis. Part I. The image acquisition process. Med Phys 2013; 40: 014301

[10] Sechopoulos I. A review of breast tomosynthesis. Part II. Image reconstruction, processing and analysis, and advanced applications. Med Phys 2013; 40: 014302

[11] Härer W, Lauritsch G, Mertelmeier T, Wiesent K. Rekonstruktive Röntgenbildgebung. Physikalische Blätter 1999; 55: 37–42

[12] Wu T, Moore RH, Rafferty EA et al. A comparison of reconstruction algorithms for breast tomosynthesis. Med Phys 2004; 31: 2636–2647

[13] Kak AC, Slaney M. Principles of Computerized Tomographic Imaging. New York: IEEE Press; 1988

[14] Lauritsch G, Haerer WH. A theoretical framework for filtered backprojection in tomosynthesis. Proc SPIE 1998; 3338: 1127–1137

[15] Mertelmeier T, Orman J, Haerer W et al. Optimizing filtered backprojection reconstruction for a breast tomosynthesis prototype device. Proc SPIE 2006; 6142: 61 420F

[16] Kunze H, Haerer W, Orman J et al. Filter determination for tomosynthesis aided by iterative reconstruction techniques. In: 9th International Meeting on Fully Three-Dimensional Image Reconstruction in Radiology and Nuclear Medicine. 2007: 309–312

[17] Ludwig J, Mertelmeier T, Kunze H. A novel approach for filtered backprojection in tomosynthesis based on filter kernels determined by iterative reconstruction techniques. In: Krupinski E (editor). Lecture Notes in Computer Science 5116, Digital Mammography, 9th International Workshop, IWDM 2008. Berlin, Heidelberg: Springer; 2008: 612–620

[18] Zhang Y, Chan H-P, Sahiner B et al. A comparative study of limited-angle cone-beam reconstruction methods for breast tomosynthesis. Med Phys 2006; 33: 3781–3795

[19] Lange K, Fessler JA. Globally convergent algorithms for maximum a posteriori transmission tomography. IEEE Trans Image Process 1995; 4: 1430–1438

[20] Ruttimann UE, Groenhuis RAJ, Webber RL. Restoration of digital multiplane tomosynthesis by a constraint iteration method. IEEE Trans Med Imaging 1984; 3: 141–148

[21] Suryanarayanan S, Karellas A, Vedantham S et al. Comparison of tomosynthesis methods used with digital mammography. Acad Radiol 2000; 7: 1085–1097

[22] Claus BEH, Eberhard JW. A new method for 3D reconstruction in digital tomosynthesis. Proc SPIE 2002; 4 684: 814–824

[23] Abdurahman S, Jerebko A, Mertelmeier T et al. Out-of-plane artifact reduction in tomosynthesis based on regression modeling and outlier detection. In: Maidment ADA, Bakic PR, Gavenonis S (editors). Lecture Notes in Computer Science 7361, Breast Imaging, 11th International Workshop, IWDM 2012. Berlin, Heidelberg: Springer; 2012: 729–736

[24] Wandell BA. Foundations of vision. Sunderland MA: Sinauer Associates; 1995

[25] Dance DR. Monte Carlo calculation of conversion factors for the estimation of mean glandular breast dose. Phys Med Biol 1990; 35: 1211–1219

[26] Dance DR, Skinner CL, Young KC et al. Additional factors for the estimation of mean glandular breast dose using the UK mammography dosimetry protocol. Phys Med Biol 2000; 45: 3225–3240

[27] Perry N, Broeders M, de Wolf C, et al (editors). European Guidelines for Quality Assurance in Breast Cancer Screening and Diagnosis, 4th Edition. Luxembourg: Office for Official Publications of the European Communities; 2006

[28] Wu X, Barnes GT, Tucker TM. Spectral dependence of glandular tissue dose in screen-film mammography. Radiology 1991; 179: 143–148

[29] Boone JM. Glandular breast dose for monoenergetic and high-energy X-ray beams: Monte Carlo assessment. Radiology 1999; 213: 23–37

[30] Boone, JM. Normalized glandular dose (DgN) coefficients for arbitrary X-ray spectra in mammography: Computer-fit values of Monte Carlo derived data. Med Phys 2002; 29: 869–875

[31] Dance DR, Young KC, van Engen RE. Estimation of mean glandular dose for breast tomosynthesis: factors for use with the UK, European and IAEA breast dosimetry protocols. Phys Med Biol 2011; 56: 453–471

[32] Sechopoulos I, Suryanarayanan S, Vedantham S et al. Computation of the glandular radiation dose in digital tomosynthesis of the breast. Med Phys 2007; 34: 221–232

[33] Bundesministerium für Umwelt, Naturschutz, Bau und Reaktorsicherheit (BMUB). Richtlinie zur Durchführung der Qualitätssicherung bei Röntgeneinrichtungen zur Untersuchung und Behandlung von Menschen nach den §§ 16 und 17 der Röntgenverordnung – Qualitätssicherungs-Richtlinie (QS-RL) [Internet]. Available at: www.bmu.de/N6 395/. Accessed May 7, 2015

[34] van Engen R, Bosmans H, Bouwman R et al. Protocol for the Quality Control of the Physical and Technical Aspects of Digital Breast Tomosynthesis Systems. Draft version 0.10, February 2013. Nijmegen: European Reference Organisation for Quality Assured Breast Screening and Diagnostic Services; 2013

Chapter 3

Clinical Evaluation of Digital Breast Tomosynthesis

3 Clinical Evaluation of Digital Breast Tomosynthesis

Berndt Michael Order, Christoph Mundhenke, Florian Vogt, Fritz K. W. Schaefer

3.1 Introduction

There is no question that full-field digital mammography continues to be the gold standard for breast imaging. Though it has lower spatial resolution than screen-film mammography, digital technology offers definite advantages in both image acquisition and display and has largely replaced screen-film mammography. The advantages of full-field digital mammography include high quantum efficiency, excellent contrast resolution, and a large dynamic range. Thus, full-field digital mammography provides the necessary diagnostic image quality, while also meeting all requirements in terms of radiation safety.[1]

However, digital technology alone cannot overcome the inherent limitation of mammography. Since mammography is a projection technique, it yields a summation image in which many anatomic structures with similar absorption characteristics or densities are superimposed. This can hamper detection and characterization of lesions. The sensitivity of mammography is greatly limited in radiographically dense breasts with an American College of Radiology (ACR) rating of 3 or 4. As a result, physiologically dense glandular structures may overlie and obscure suspicious changes such as focal lesions or architectural distortions. Moreover, conventional projection mammograms often yield false-positive findings, owing to summation effects. This occurs when normal breast structures are superimposed in the path of the X-ray beam, creating an overlap density that requires further evaluation by supplementary methods such as breast ultrasonography or special views.

Digital breast tomosynthesis (DBT) attempts to add information and overcome the limitations of mammography. The reconstruction of tomographic image slices of the breast eliminates summation effects and improves the detectability of focal lesions. Various questions must be addressed in order to define the clinical role of DBT as accurately as possible and establish guidelines for its use. A number of studies have focused on several key issues:

- Does tomosynthesis add information to that supplied by digital mammography?
- Can tomosynthesis replace additional mammographic views?
- Can tomosynthesis replace mammography?

Another issue to be considered is radiation exposure. The ultimate goal is clear: to achieve greater diagnostic accuracy at a lower dose. This underscores the need to achieve higher sensitivity and specificity in DBT than in standard two-view mammography. Progress must be gradual, however, for two reasons. First, the technical evolution of DBT is far from complete; and second, more extensive clinical experience and ongoing training in the evaluation of tomosynthesis are needed in order to fully establish the diagnostic potential of this technology.

3.2 Mammography versus Mammography Plus Tomosynthesis

Various studies have already been done to determine whether tomosynthesis can add information to that provided by digital mammography. In each of these studies, mammography alone was compared with a combination of mammography and tomosynthesis. In an initial clinical study, Poplack et al studied a cohort of 98 women with abnormal digital screening mammograms who required recall.[2] In all patients, a total of 11 low-dose exposures were taken in a 19-second scan and were reconstructed into tomosynthesis images. The study confirmed that the rate of recall based on findings detected on screening could have been reduced by 40% by the addition of tomosynthesis. The benefits of tomosynthesis over mammography resulted from the more accurate evaluation of lesion margins and the minimization of summation effects from overlapping tissues. Tomosynthesis improved accuracy in the detection or exclusion of architectural distortions, asymmetries, and focal lesions (masses) (**Fig. 3.1**).

Tomosynthesis did not prove helpful for the morphologic analysis of suspicious microcalcifications in this study. The authors concluded that, for evaluation of calcifications, the image quality from tomosynthesis was inferior to that of full-field digital mammography. This may have resulted from motion artifacts or the low reconstructed slice thickness. A key limitation in this study, however, was the small number of cases.

Building on the encouraging initial results, further studies were undertaken in larger groups of patients.[3,4] The studies differ primarily in their inclusion criteria, number of projection images acquired, and study design.

A large multicenter study with a total of 27 readers compared the diagnostic accuracy of two-view mammography alone or combined with two-view tomosynthesis.[5] Two groups were formed from the study population of more than 1,000 women. Study 1 comprised 312 cases with a total of 48 cancers and images read by 12 radiologists. The readers determined only whether an abnormality requiring recall was present or absent. In study 2 (310 cases, 51 cancers, 15 radiologists), the lesion type and location were also recorded.

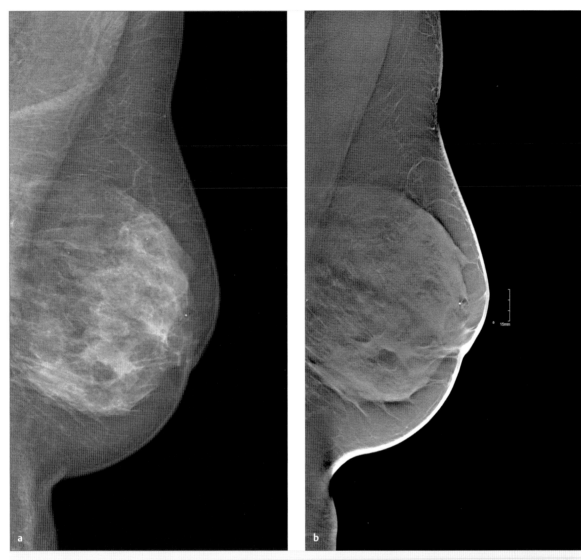

Fig. 3.1 A 1-cm spiculated mass is located approximately 3.5 cm from the nipple in the left breast. The lesion is depicted more clearly by DBT than mammography. Histology identified the lesion as invasive lobular carcinoma. **(a)** Digital mammogram of the left breast, mediolateral oblique (MLO) projection. **(b)** DBT of the left breast, MLO projection.

All 27 radiologists found that the addition of tomosynthesis improved diagnostic accuracy, while the recall rates for individual readers were reduced by between 6 and 67%. The addition of tomosynthesis was particularly effective in improving the detection of invasive cancers, whereas it provided little gain in the detection of in situ cancers. Based on their results, the authors concluded that the addition of tomosynthesis to digital mammography improves diagnostic accuracy and significantly reduces the recall rates for noncancer cases.

In summary, all studies in patients with suspicious mammograms have shown that tomosynthesis provides a diagnostic gain when used as an adjunct to mammogra- phy. It is unclear from the studies whether tomosynthesis could also be used effectively in an unselected population and in an algorithm that includes double reading.

This question was addressed in the Oslo Tomosynthesis Screening Trial.[6] A total of 12,621 women from a nation- wide screening program in Norway underwent bilateral mammography in the craniocaudal (CC) and MLO projec- tions plus bilateral tomosynthesis in the CC and MLO pro- jections. Both the conventional and tomosynthesis im- ages were acquired during a single breast compression per view. Four experienced radiologists read the images in four different study arms:

- Two-dimensional (2D) mammography alone.

- 2D mammography plus computer-aided detection (CAD).
- 2D mammography plus tomosynthesis.
- Synthesized 2D images reconstructed from the tomosynthesis data, plus three-dimensional (3D) tomosynthesis.

All examinations that were rated suspicious in one of the study arms were subsequently discussed in a consensus meeting and referred for recall if necessary.

The addition of tomosynthesis increased the recall rate: 365 women with suspicious mammographic findings were recalled, compared with 463 women with suspicious findings by mammography or tomosynthesis. This led to a 30% increase in the cancer-detection rate in the study arms with adjunctive tomosynthesis. In absolute terms, the cancer-detection rates were 0.71% with mammography alone (7.1 cancers per 1,000 women screened) and 0.94% in the tomosynthesis groups. Most of the additional cancers detected by tomosynthesis were node-negative invasive tumors. The cancer-detection rate relative to the total number of recalls was approximately 25% in both study groups, with or without tomosynthesis.

Besides diagnostic accuracy, this study also addressed two other important aspects. The average reading time for 2D mammography was 48 seconds per reading, but this increased to 89 seconds when tomosynthesis was added. This doubling of the reading time would significantly increase the workload in a screening program. The second aspect is radiation exposure. The average parenchymal dose was 1.58 ± 0.61 milligray (mGy) for mammography, 1.95 ± 0.58 mGy for tomosynthesis, and 3.52 ± 1.08 mGy for the combination of mammography and tomosynthesis.

Another study was conducted in a total screening population of 13,158 women.[7] All patients underwent two-view digital mammography, and 6,100 of the women underwent digital mammography plus two-view DBT. The cancer-detection rates in the two groups were compared. In contrast to the study by Skaane et al,[6] the recall rate in the DBT group, at 8.5%, was lower than in patients receiving mammography alone (12%). The cancer-detection rate was 0.52% with mammography alone versus 0.57% with mammography plus tomosynthesis ($P = 0.70$).

Recently, Friedewald et al[8] published a retrospective analysis of screening performance metrics from 13 sites in the United States of America, using mixed models adjusting for site as a random effect. A total of 281,187 digital mammographies and 173,663 combined examinations (digital mammography plus tomosynthesis) were evaluated. Model-adjusted rates per 1,000 screens resulted in a recall rate of 107 with digital mammography versus 91 for digital mammography plus tomosynthesis. The number of biopsies increased by 1.3 per 1,000 screens (18.1 with digital mammography versus 19.3 with digital mammography plus tomosynthesis). Cancer detection

significantly increased from 0.42% with digital mammography to 0.54% for digital mammography plus tomosynthesis. This large multicenter study confirmed the results of the previous studies and demonstrated that the addition of tomosynthesis to digital mammography resulted in a decreased recall rate and an increased cancer-detection rate.

In summary, all the studies confirm that in both selected and screened populations, the addition of tomosynthesis to digital mammography led to improved diagnostic accuracy and an increase in cancer-detection rates. A number of questions remain to be answered, however. In particular, data are needed that can show whether tomosynthesis actually requires two views when used as an adjunct to mammography. Because tomosynthesis supplies 3D information, one-view tomosynthesis may be sufficient. Further large studies are needed to resolve this issue.

3.3 Tomosynthesis versus Additional Mammographic Views

The routine combination of two-view mammograms with one- or two-view tomosynthesis increases diagnostic accuracy but also raises concerns about radiation safety. It is common in routine clinical settings, however, for two-view mammograms to yield equivocal results that require further evaluation by additional views (e.g., spot compression and microfocus magnification views). This raises the question of whether tomosynthesis could be useful in these cases and whether it is equivalent or even superior to additional mammographic views (**Fig. 3.2**).

In 2010, Hakim and his group compared the value of adjunctive digital tomosynthesis with additional mammographic views in the characterization of known mammographic masses, architectural distortions, and asymmetries.[9] Four experienced radiologists interpreted full-field digital mammograms aided by additional views or DBT images, in 25 women. The radiologists were asked to determine which combination yielded the best diagnostic accuracy.

In 50% of the ratings, the radiologists perceived the combination of full-field digital mammography plus DBT to be diagnostically superior to full-field digital mammography plus additional views. Both combinations were rated equivalent in 31% of cases, and the addition of DBT was rated as inferior to additional mammographic views in 19%. Over all the readers, 92% of the ratings for known breast cancer cases and 50% of the ratings for known high-risk lesions were classified as BI-RADS 4 or 5. The authors concluded that DBT provided an alternative to additional mammographic views for the characterization

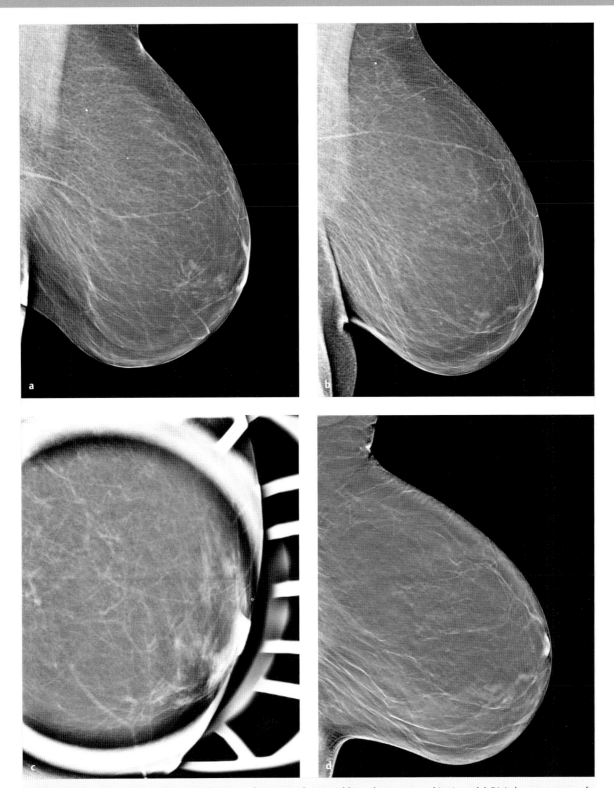

Fig. 3.2 Illustrative case in which tomosynthesis is at least equivalent to additional mammographic views. **(a)** Digital mammogram of the left breast in the MLO projection shows a new 2.5-cm subareolar architectural distortion that has no correlate in the CC view. Classified as BI-RADS 4. **(b)** Digital mammogram of the left breast, ML projection. A focal lesion is not visible in this view. **(c)** Digital spot compression view of the left breast, MLO projection. A focal lesion is not visible in this view. **(d)** Single slice from a 3D tomosynthesis data set of the left breast, MLO projection. This image positively identifies the suspicious area as a summation effect caused by residual parenchyma and superimposed vessels. Based on this finding, the left breast was reclassified as BI-RADS 2.

of focal abnormalities detected in two-view mammograms.

Another study compared DBT with mammographic spot views in the characterization of 67 breast masses as benign or malignant.[10] Four radiologists rated the images for mass visibility, likelihood of malignancy, and BI-RADS classification. The mass visibility ratings were slightly better with DBT. The four readers detected seven additional cancers with DBT, although five of the biopsies yielded a benign result (false-positive biopsy recommendations). The authors concluded that both methods were equivalent for the characterization of breast masses.

In the largest study on this topic published to date, eight radiologists reviewed a series of 217 lesions in 182 patients.[11] Seventy-two of the lesions (33%) were cancers and 145 (67%) were benign. All eight readers achieved better results with tomosynthesis than with mammographic spot views (by receiver operating characteristic [ROC] curve analysis) in the detection of malignant lesions. With tomosynthesis, more cancers were classified as BI-RADS 5 with no decrease in specificity. The false-positive rate for all lesions classified as BI-RADS 4 or 5 decreased from 57% to 48% ($P < 0.01$) with tomosynthesis, with no change in sensitivity. The authors concluded that tomosynthesis significantly improved diagnostic accuracy for equivocal focal lesions, compared with mammographic spot views.

In all studies to date comparing DBT and spot compression views, tomosynthesis was found to be at least equivalent to the additional views. This means that DBT may be considered a preferred imaging technique for the further evaluation of suspicious mammographic lesions in routine clinical settings. It should be added, however, that this statement applies only to masses, architectural distortions, and asymmetries, because suspicious microcalcifications were not investigated in most studies.

However, microcalcifications are a finding of very great clinical importance, especially for the detection of ductal carcinoma in situ (DCIS). They are also a challenge to imaging. Numerous studies have shown that digital mammography is superior to screen-film mammography in the detection of microcalcifications. The question of whether tomosynthesis can detect microcalcifications with comparable sensitivity cannot be definitively answered at present.

An initial study by Spangler et al in 2011 dealt with the detection and classification of microcalcifications by digital tomosynthesis compared with digital mammography.[12] One hundred examinations were performed, using both full-field digital mammography and tomosynthesis.

The series included 20 histologically confirmed cancers, 40 histologically confirmed benign calcifications, and 40 randomly selected negative screening studies. Five radiologists reviewed the images in a multireader setting. The sensitivity for detecting calcifications was 84% for full-field digital mammography and 75% for digital tomosynthesis. The two methods had comparable performance as measured by the ROC analysis of BI-RADS scores (full-field digital mammography: ROC area under the curve [AUC] = 0.76, standard deviation [SD] = 0.03; digital tomosynthesis: ROC AUC = 0.72, SD = 0.04).

However, a similar study by Kopans et al found that DBT was superior to conventional mammography.[13] A total of 119 cases with suspicious microcalcifications were reviewed in this study. Only the MLO view was available for digital tomosynthesis, while both the MLO and CC views were available for conventional mammograms. In 41.6% of cases, the readers stated that calcifications were seen with better clarity on digital tomosynthesis. Both methods were comparable in 50.4% of cases, and conventional mammography was felt to be superior in 8% of cases. Another study also found that DBT was superior to mammography in the detection of microcalcifications.[14] The difference between the two methods was greater for less experienced readers than for readers with 10 or more years' experience in breast imaging.

In most studies, then, tomosynthesis has shown excellent results in the detection of microcalcifications (**Fig. 3.3**). With the 3D information supplied by tomosynthesis, the spatial distribution of the calcifications can be accurately evaluated. Advantages include the positive identification of cutaneous calcifications and the confident detection of linear intraductal spread. When it comes to the assessment of microcalcification morphology, however, 3D tomosynthesis is inferior to standard 2D mammography and microfocus magnification views.

In summary, studies to date have reported varying results in the detection and characterization of microcalcifications. The advantages of nonsuperimposed images and accurate spatial localization must be weighed against the potential disadvantages of partial-volume effects and motion artifacts. Also, the studies have used systems that vary in their acquisition parameters, image postprocessing, and size of the detector elements. These differences can be particularly significant in the detection of microcalcifications. Consequently, the results of different studies cannot be directly compared with one another. Larger studies are needed before it is possible to definitively assess the sensitivity and specificity of DBT in the detection and characterization of breast microcalcifications.

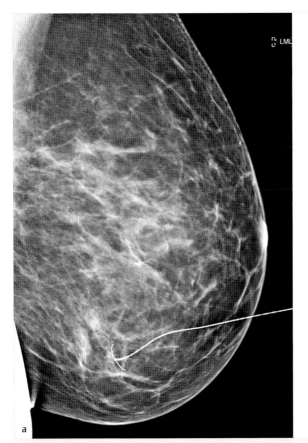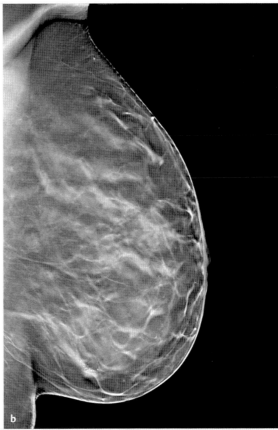

Fig. 3.3 Histologically confirmed high-grade ductal carcinoma in situ. **(a)** Digital mammogram of the left breast, ML projection with a localization wire in place. A cluster of pleomorphic microcalcifications, already localized with the wire, is visible in the lower inner quadrant of the breast, 9.5 cm from the nipple. Classified as BI-RADS 5. **(b)** Single slice from a 3D tomosynthesis data set of the left breast, MLO projection before wire insertion. The calcifications are displayed with excellent clarity, and their arrangement and configuration identify them as ductal calcifications. Classified as BI-RADS 5.

3.4 Mammography versus Tomosynthesis

To answer the question of whether tomosynthesis can replace mammography, studies are needed in which mammography and DBT are evaluated separately.

Andersson et al conducted a pilot study in 40 women with subtle signs of breast cancer on screening mammography, or symptomatic women with negative mammographic findings but suspicious findings on ultrasonography.[15] The authors compared breast cancer visibility in one-view tomosynthesis with that in one- and two-view full-field digital mammography. Tomosynthesis was performed in the same orientation as the mammographic image in which the tumor was least visible or not visible. Otherwise tomosynthesis was performed in the standard MLO view. Two radiologists interpreted the mammograms and DBT images in a consensus reading.

Cancer visibility was classified into four categories, and BI-RADS scores were also assigned. In 22 of 40 cases, the cancers were rated as more visible on tomosynthesis compared with one-view mammography. When tomosynthesis was compared with two-view mammography, cancer visibility on DBT was rated better in 11 of 40 cases ($P < 0.01$). When one-view mammography was compared with tomosynthesis, 21 patients were upgraded to a higher BI-RADS category. Comparing two-view mammography with tomosynthesis, 12 patients were upgraded on BI-RADS classification. Again, the differences were statistically significant. Microcalcification analysis by tomosynthesis was correct only in terms of distribution and cluster shape; tomosynthesis was less effective for the morphologic analysis of individual particles. Despite this limitation, the authors concluded that tomosynthesis provided significantly better tumor visibility and a more accurate BI-RADS classification than digital mammography.

Building on the results of this pilot study, additional studies were done to assess the role of DBT in relation to mammography. In one prospective study, two-view tomosynthesis was performed as an adjunct in 513 women with an abnormal screening mammogram (two-view full-field digital mammography) or with clinical symptoms.[16] The full-field mammograms and DBT images were separately and prospectively classified according to BI-RADS criteria. A total of 112 cancers were detected. Tomosynthesis and full-field mammography were each able to detect 104 cancers and were each false negative in eight cases (7%). In the false-negative mammographic cases, four of the tumors were detected by ultrasonography, two by magnetic resonance imaging, one by recall after breast tomosynthesis interpretation, and one only after mastectomy. The sensitivity of both techniques for the detection of breast cancer was 92.9%. The specificities of mammography and tomosynthesis were 86.1% and 84.4%, respectively ($P = 0.37$). It should be added, however, that two cancers were missed by tomosynthesis, owing to technical problems (patient motion, positioning errors).

Wallis et al compared the diagnostic accuracy of 2D full-field mammography with that of two-view (mediolateral [ML] and CC) and one-view (MLO) tomosynthesis, in an interobserver study of 220 women.[14] The diagnostic accuracy of 2D full-field mammography was significantly poorer than that of two-view tomosynthesis (ROC AUC = 0.772 for 2D mammography, ROC AUC = 0.851 for tomosynthesis). No significant difference was found between 2D mammography (AUC = 0.774) and one-view tomosynthesis (AUC = 0.775). This suggests that one-view tomosynthesis (in the MLO projection) is comparable to two-view full-field digital mammography.

Another study by Gennaro et al enrolled 200 women who had at least one breast lesion classified by mammography and/or ultrasonography as doubtful, suspicious, or probably malignant.[17] In addition to the two-view mammograms already available, tomosynthesis was performed in the MLO projection. The images were scored separately by six radiologists, using BI-RADS criteria. Based on ROC analysis, the results did not show a significant difference between the two methods. The authors concluded that one-view tomosynthesis was not inferior to two-view digital mammography.

All the studies cited thus far have one serious limitation: They were done mainly in women with mammographic abnormalities. This creates a selection bias that favors mammography and gives no information about diagnostic performance in an unselected screening population. This question is addressed by the Malmö Breast Tomosynthesis Screening Trial. The goal of the trial is to enroll 15,000 women from a population-based screening program, who will undergo two-view digital mammography in addition to one-view tomosynthesis. The number of breast cancers detected by digital mammography alone will be compared with the number detected by one-view tomosynthesis without simultaneous consideration of the mammographic findings. The trial was started in 2010, and enrollment of the participants should be completed in 2015. The results of the study will answer the question of whether one-view tomosynthesis can reliably replace two-view screening mammography.

Given the remaining uncertainty about the diagnostic accuracy of tomosynthesis in detecting microcalcifications on the one hand, and the superiority of tomosynthesis for mass detection on the other, it might be effective to combine one-view mammography with complementary-view tomosynthesis. Gennaro et al tried this approach in 463 breasts with a total of 348 lesions, consisting of 77 cancers and 271 benign lesions.[17] A total of six radiologists with at least 7 years' experience in breast imaging conducted a per-lesion analysis.

The combination of one-view DBT (MLO) with one-view digital mammography (CC) was superior to standard two-view digital mammography in both the detection and characterization of lesions: 60% of the lesions were correctly detected with mammography alone versus 66.5% of the lesions with DBT plus mammography in complementary views ($P < 0.0001$). The difference in lesion characterization was greatest for benign lesions: 42.4% of benign lesions were correctly characterized in the study arm with DBT, as opposed to 34.4% with two-view mammography alone ($P < 0.0001$).

3.5 Summary

Tomosynthesis is a new technique of breast imaging that has added clinically relevant information in all larger studies and has proven equal or even superior to mammography in available comparative studies. The most important studies have been published only in the last 3 years, and the results of additional large studies are not yet available. It will therefore be several years before tomosynthesis can be incorporated into clinically relevant guidelines and mammographic screening.

For the time being, digital breast tomography can be used for routine investigation of equivocal mammographic findings. There are not yet sufficient data available to recommend tomosynthesis as a replacement for mammography. The combination of one-view mammography and one-view tomosynthesis can be used in selected cases, such as investigational settings and patients with significant fibrocystic breast changes.

3.6 References

[1] Schulz-Wendtland R, Fuchsjäger M, Wacker T et al. Digital mammography: an update. Eur J Radiol 2009; 72: 258–265

[2] Poplack SP, Tosteson TD, Kogel CA et al. Digital breast tomosynthesis: initial experience in 98 women with abnormal digital screening mammography. AJR Am J Roentgenol 2007; 189: 616–623

[3] Svahn TM, Chakraborty DP, Ikeda D. Breast tomosynthesis and digital mammography: a comparison of diagnostic accuracy. Br J Radiol 2012; 85: e1074–e1082

[4] Michell MJ, Iqbal A, Wasan RK et al. A comparison of the accuracy of film-screen mammography, full-field digital mammography and digital breast tomosynthesis. Clin Radiol 2012; 67: 976–981

[5] Rafferty EA, Park JM, Philpotts LE et al. Assessing radiologist performance using combined digital mammography and breast tomosynthesis compared with digital mammography alone: results of a multicenter, multireader trial. Radiology 2013; 266:104–113

[6] Skaane P, Bandos AI, Gullien R et al. Prospective trial comparing full-field digital mammography (FFDM) versus combined FFDM and tomosynthesis in a population-based screening programme using independent double reading with arbitration. Eur Radiol 2013; 23: 2061–2071

[7] Haas BM, Kalra V, Geisel J et al. Comparison of tomosynthesis plus digital mammography and digital mammography alone for breast cancer screening. Radiology 2013; 269: 694–700

[8] Friedewald SM, Rafferty EA, Rose SL et al. Breast cancer screening using tomosynthesis in combination with digital mammography. JAMA 2014; 24: 2499–2507

[9] Hakim CM, Chough DM, Ganott MA et al. Digital breast tomosynthesis in the diagnostic environment: A subjective side-by-side review. AJR Am J Roentgenol 2010; 195: 172–176

[10] Noroozian M, Hadjiiski L, Rahnama-Moghadam S et al. Digital breast tomosynthesis is comparable to mammographic spot views for mass characterization. Radiology 2012; 262: 61–68

[11] Zuley ML, Bandos AI, Ganott MA et al. Digital breast tomosynthesis versus supplemental diagnostic mammographic views for evaluation of noncalcified breast lesions. Radiology 2013; 266: 89–95

[12] Spangler ML, Zuley ML, Sumkin JA et al. Detection and classification of calcifications on digital breast tomosynthesis and 2D digital mammography: a comparison. AJR Am J Roentgenol 2011; 196: 320–324

[13] Kopans D, Gavenonis S, Halpern E et al. Calcifications in the breast and digital breast tomosynthesis. Breast J 2011; 17: 638–644

[14] Wallis MG, Moa E, Zanca F et al. Two-view and single-view tomosynthesis versus full-field digital mammography: high-resolution X-ray imaging observer study. Radiology 2012; 262: 788–796

[15] Andersson I, Ikeda DM, Zackrisson S. Breast tomosynthesis and digital mammography: a comparison of breast cancer visibility and BIRADS classification in a population of cancers with subtle mammographic findings. Eur Radiol 2008; 18: 2817–2825

[16] Teertstra HJ, Loo CE, van den Bosch MAAJ et al. Breast tomosynthesis in clinical practice: initial results. Eur Radiol 2010; 20: 16–24

[17] Gennaro G, Toledano A, di Maggio C et al. Digital breast tomosynthesis versus digital mammography: a clinical performance study. Eur Radiol 2010; 20: 1545–1553

Chapter 4

Innovations and Future Developments

4

4 Innovations and Future Developments

Fritz K. W. Schaefer and Joerg Barkhausen

4.1 Introduction

Tomosynthesis is still a relatively new technology, and its technical evolution is far from complete. Compared to mammography, it still has great potential for advances in image reconstruction and postprocessing, as well as new clinical applications. Some of the techniques described in this chapter are still conceptual, some exist as prototypes, and some are already in clinical use. In all cases, however, the benefits of these techniques have not yet been adequately evaluated for routine clinical use, and it is still too early to draw definite conclusions.

4.2 Synthesized Digital Two-dimensional Mammography

New techniques are currently being developed for the reconstruction of conventional mammograms from a three-dimensional (3D) tomosynthesis data set (**Fig. 4.1**). Comparison of a 3D tomosynthesis data set and the corresponding slices with digital or even analog mammography poses a significant challenge. It is therefore desirable not only to reconstruct sectional images from the digital breast tomosynthesis (DBT) projections but also to generate a summation image that is comparable to a mammo-

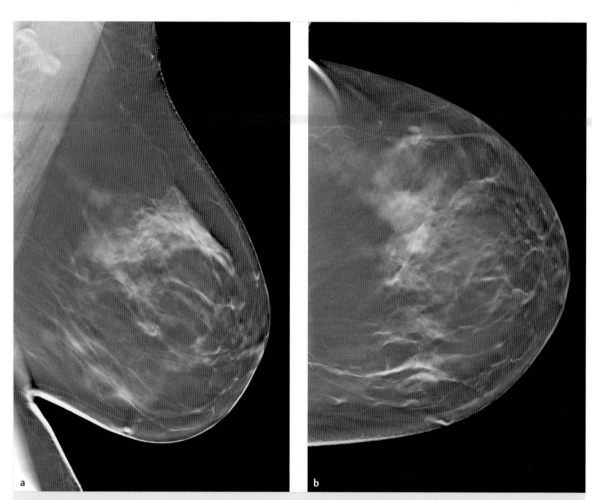

Fig. 4.1 Tubular breast cancer, confirmed histologically by core-needle biopsy. (Image data were provided courtesy of M. Sonnenschein, MD, Bern, Switzerland.) **(a)** 3D tomosynthesis of the left breast, mediolateral oblique (MLO) projection: 14-mm spiculated lesion at the 1 o'clock position. **(b)** 3D tomosynthesis of the left breast, craniocaudal (CC) projection: 14-mm spiculated lesion at the 1 o'clock position.

continued ▶

gram. With this technique, called synthesized digital two-dimensional (2D) mammography ("c-view"), both sectional images and mammograms for comparison with prior images can be reconstructed from a DBT data set, without additional radiation exposure.

On initial viewing, the synthesized 2D image has a notably artificial appearance. The skin is markedly thickened in comparison with conventional mammograms, and this finding should not be mistaken for edema. There is also a marked accentuation of tissue contrasts, which may, for example, cause microcalcifications to appear more prominent. A first study on the performance of reconstructed 2D images in combination with DBT versus full-field digital mammography (FFDM) combined with DBT was published by Skaane et al in 2014.[1] Using the most recent version of synthetically reconstructed 2D images, the cancer-detection rate was 7.8/1,000 for FFDM plus DBT versus 7.7/1,000 for reconstructed 2D images plus DBT, and the false-positive rate was 4.6% for FFDM plus DBT versus 4.5% for the current version of reconstructed 2D images plus DBT. The authors concluded that the combination of the current reconstructed 2D images plus DBT performed comparably to FFDM plus DBT and may be adequate for routine clinical use when interpreting screening mammograms.[1]

4.3 Computer-aided Detection in Tomosynthesis

Computer-aided detection (CAD) systems for digital mammography have been in development for 20 years and have been commercially available for digital mammography for approximately 10 years. These systems

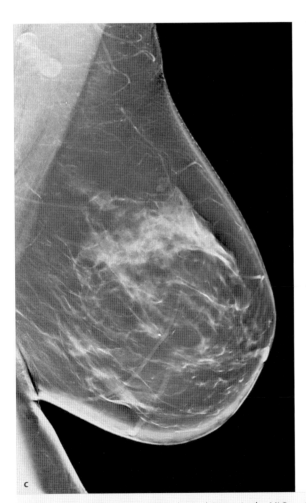
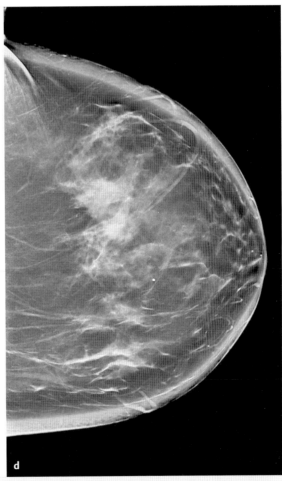

Fig. 4.1 (continued) **(c)** Summation (c-view) image in the MLO projection, synthesized from the tomosynthesis data set. In overall appearance, the image closely resembles a conventional digital mammogram. **(d)** Summation (c-view) image in the CC projection, synthesized from the tomosynthesis data set. The image closely resembles a conventional digital mammogram. The spiculated mass is visualized but is more difficult to detect compared with 3D tomosynthesis. However, the image does facilitate comparison with prior images.

cannot be applied to tomosynthesis without modifications, however: While the acquired image slices, with their extremely large data volumes, open new possibilities for image postprocessing, they also present new challenges. Thus, for detection of breast masses, CAD systems may work with projection images, reconstructed slices, or a combination of projection images and slices.

A recent study used a CAD system focused on 2D images for mass detection in tomosynthesis.[2] With this approach, it has proven helpful to assemble multiple DBT slices into a thicker slab, as this produces images that are more similar to standard mammograms. This algorithm was tested in 192 patients, and the best results were achieved with a slab thickness of 15 mm.

Besides mass detection, CAD systems could also be used for characterization of lesions by methods such as volumetric segmentation. A prototype system of this kind is available and was successfully tested on experimental data sets.[3] Adequate experience with clinical data sets is not yet available, however.

CAD systems could also be used in tomosynthesis for the detection of microcalcifications. The first prototype software for this application was tested on 72 DBT data sets with histologically confirmed microcalcification clusters (17 cancers, 55 benign lesions). The study succeeded in developing a more advanced algorithm, but the average number of false positives was 3.4 per DBT data set, with a sensitivity of only 85%.[4] This false-positive rate is still too high for clinical use.

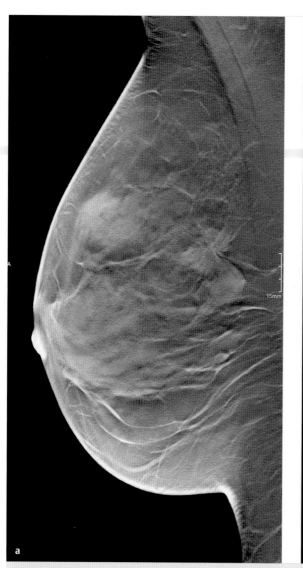
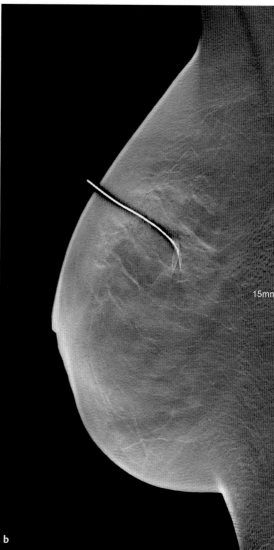

Fig. 4.2 Tomosynthesis data set in the MLO projection, before and after wire localization of a mass. **(a)** Image slice before wire localization. A suspicious spiculated mass is visible. **(b)** Image slice after wire localization of the mass. The wire shaft is sharply defined, but its tip is ill-defined and obscured by artifacts.

continued ▶

4.4 Tomosynthesis-guided Interventions

Numerous studies have shown that digital tomosynthesis improves lesion detection and characterization. This suggests that the additional information supplied by DBT may be useful for guiding breast biopsies or localizing suspicious breast changes. Any improvement in imaging requires corresponding advances in biopsy techniques. A first step in this direction is using DBT to check the placement of localization wires (**Fig. 4.2**).

However, for lesions that are not visualized with other imaging modalities, DBT-guided interventions would be desirable. Freer et al performed DBT-guided needle local-izations using a commercially available system, in 36 architectural distortions that were only visible with tomosynthesis.[5] The procedure was technically successful in all patients and the histological results showed 17 malignant lesions, 5 high-risk lesions, and 14 benign lesions. The authors concluded that DBT-guided needle localization is feasible and accurate. Additionally, the results indicate that a suspicious architectural distortion that is only visible with DBT has a high lesion-level positive predictive value of 47% for malignancy.[5]

The system used in this study was marketed in 2013 and additionally enables vacuum and core-needle biopsies under 3D tomosynthesis guidance. The biopsy unit is mounted on the compression device, and the intervention can be performed with the patient sitting or lying

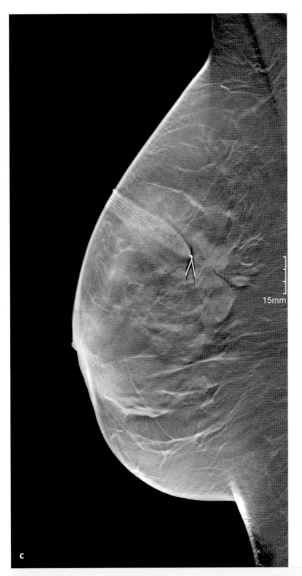
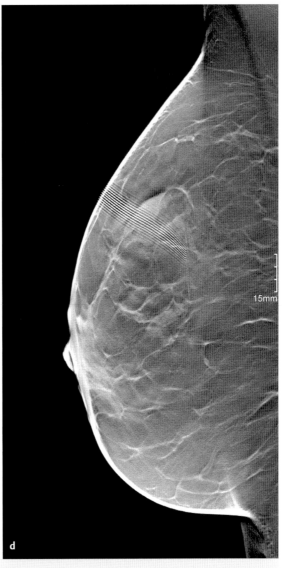

Fig. 4.2 (continued) **(c)** Image slice at a deeper level after wire localization of the mass. The wire tip is sharply defined and located approximately 5 mm from the lesion. Overshoot artifacts are visible along the wire shaft. **(d)** Image slice at an even deeper level, after wire localization of the mass. The artifacts have spread out in a fan-shaped pattern.

down. The procedure lasts only a few minutes, and initial experience indicates that it is very well tolerated.

Schrading et al compared the clinical performance of prone stereotactic vacuum-assisted biopsy (VAB) with DBT-guided VAB in 205 patients with 216 mammographic findings.[6] Prone stereotactic VAB was performed in 159 patients with 165 target lesions, whereas DBT-guided VAB was performed in 46 patients with 51 target lesions. The technical success rate was 100% with DBT and 93% using stereotactic guidance, with a shorter mean intervention time in the DBT group (13 versus 29 minutes). DBT was especially helpful in low-contrast lesions and increased the number of these lesions being biopsied successfully, compared to stereotactic guidance. The authors concluded that the clinical performance of DBT VAB was significantly superior to stereotactic guidance and may replace stereotactic VAB for routine use in all patients with abnormal mammographic findings.[6]

However, unlike breast tissue, biopsy needles and localization wires are high-contrast objects that may cause artifacts.[7] These artifacts are influenced by the thickness of the foreign materials, their position and orientation, and the reconstruction algorithms. Minimizing these artifacts (e.g., by special image-reconstruction techniques) to maintain optimum visualization of small target lesions throughout the intervention will become an important goal in the years ahead.

4.5 Contrast-enhanced Tomosynthesis

A major advantage of tomosynthesis over conventional mammography is its ability to provide nonsuperimposed views of intramammary structures. However, the differentiation of masses from breast tissue is only possible if they have different densities, and these differences tend to be smallest in radiographically dense breasts. Even tomosynthesis, therefore, is limited in its ability to detect focal lesions.

For this reason, it would be desirable to enhance density differences between masses and glandular tissue during tomosynthesis. One way to do this is by intravenous contrast administration, which could highlight the distinctive perfusion and enhancement characteristics of tumors.

However, because the expected density differences are relatively small, contrast-enhanced tomosynthesis must be combined with techniques that can amplify low object contrast, to produce maximum image contrast. One possible solution would be spectral tomosynthesis.[8]

A technically simpler approach to this problem is to take two exposures, using a "dual-energy" technique. The first exposure is taken at a low kilovoltage below the k-edge of iodine (33 kV), and a higher tube voltage is used for the second exposure. A variant of this technique,

which requires just one exposure, employs an extremely fast detector that detects all X-ray quanta below a threshold of 33 kV, for example, and all X-ray quanta above that level, resulting in one low-energy image and one high-energy image. When the two images are then subtracted, iodine is detected with exquisite sensitivity, resulting in a high degree of iodinated contrast enhancement.

In an initial study in 21 patients with various breast lesions (Breast Imaging Reporting and Data System [BI-RADS] 4 or higher), spectral tomosynthesis was performed before, 120 seconds after, and 480 seconds after the intravenous administration of 1 mL of iodinated contrast agent per kilogram of body weight. Contrast-enhanced magnetic resonance imaging (MRI) was used as a reference standard. The study showed that the contrast agent kinetics could be assessed using spectral tomosynthesis. Moreover, the signal intensity–time curves in spectral tomosynthesis were comparable to those in contrast-enhanced MRI.[9]

On the other hand, the analysis of contrast agent kinetics by DBT at different times after contrast administration requires greater radiation exposure than standard imaging. For this reason, all possibilities for dose optimization should be exhausted before clinical trials of this procedure are instituted in large numbers of patients.

4.6 References

[1] Skaane P, Bandos AI, Eben EB et al. Two-view digital breast tomosynthesis screening with synthetically reconstructed projection images: comparison with digital breast tomosynthesis with full-field digital mammographic images. Radiology 2014; 271(3): 655–663

[2] van Schie G, Wallis MG, Leifland K et al. Mass detection in reconstructed digital breast tomosynthesis volumes with a computeraided detection system trained on 2D mammograms. Med Phys 2013; 40: 041 902

[3] Wittenberg T, Wagner F, Gryanik A. Towards a computer assisted diagnosis system for digital breast tomosynthesis. Biomed Tech 2012; 57 (suppl 1)

[4] Sahiner B, Chan HP, Hadjiiski LM et al. Computer-aided detection of clustered microcalcifications in digital breast tomosynthesis: a 3D approach. Med Phys 2012; 39: 28–39

[5] Freer PE, Niell B, Rafferty EA. Preoperative tomosynthesis-guided needle localization of mammographically and sonographically occult breast lesions. Radiology 2015; 275(2): 377–383

[6] Schrading S, Distelmaier M, Dirrichs T et al. Digital breast tomosynthesis-guided vacuum-assisted breast biopsy: initial experiences and comparison with prone stereotactic vacuum-assisted biopsy; Radiology 2015; 274(3): 654–662

[7] Wu T, Moore RH, Kopans DB. Voting strategy for artifact reduction in digital breast tomosynthesis. Med Phys 2006; 33: 2461–2471

[8] Fredenberg E, Hemmendorff M, Cederström B et al. Contrast-enhanced spectral mammography with a photon-counting detector. Med Phys 2010; 37: 2017–2029

[9] Froeling V, Diekmann F, Renz DM et al. Correlation of contrast agent kinetics between iodinated contrast-enhanced spectral tomosynthesis and gadolinium-enhanced MRI of breast lesions. Eur Radiol 2013; 23: 1528–1536

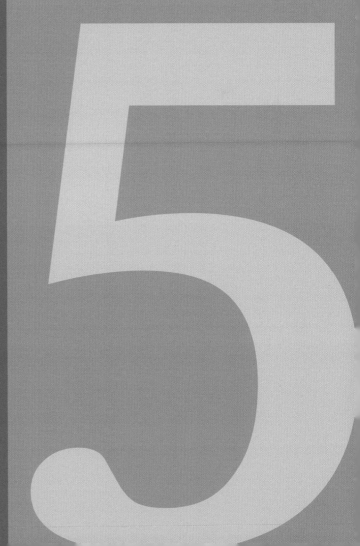

Chapter 5

Illustrative Case Reports

5 Illustrative Case Reports

Kristin Baumann, Dorothea Fischer, Isabell Grande-Nagel, Smaragda Kapsimalakou, Berndt Michael Order, Fritz K. W. Schaefer

5.1 Introduction

The case reports in this chapter cover a range of findings that demonstrate both the capabilities and limitations of digital breast tomography. Cases imaged by multiple modalities are included, to permit a direct comparison of the findings. Note that all of the modalities in these cases were not necessary for a complete work-up, which did not follow a standard algorithm. There are several reasons why comprehensive images were available for selected cases: Some patients had already undergone various tests elsewhere before adjunctive tomosynthesis was performed, during interventional planning to establish their lesion histology. Other patients underwent more imaging studies than were strictly necessary because they were participants in clinical trials.

As in the everyday practice of breast imaging, the cases are not arranged by topics. Each case is illustrated by selected, representative tomosynthesis image slices. In some cases, however, it is easier to detect lesions by scrolling through an image stack. Video sequences for nearly half the cases have been made available online, and it is always worthwhile to view the sequences that cover a complete digital breast tomosynthesis (DBT) data set.

5.2 Cases

5.2.1 Case 1

History

A 72-year-old woman with a family history of breast cancer. For several months, she has noticed skin dimpling at the 3 o'clock position in the left breast, with increasing local firmness. Clinical examination reveals a typical plateau sign 9 cm lateral to the nipple and a mass of approximately 2 cm fixed to the chest wall.

Mammography

Left breast: American College of Radiology (ACR) 3. Skin retraction is noted in the upper outer quadrant of the left breast, 9 cm from the nipple, also a 2.1-cm spiculated mass with ill-defined margins. Classified as Breast Imaging Reporting and Data System (BI-RADS) 5 (**Fig. 5.1a, b**).

DBT

Tomosynthesis views of the left breast in the craniocaudal (CC) and mediolateral oblique (MLO) projections demonstrate a spiculated mass and skin retraction. The lesion appears less dense in the CC view than on mammograms. Classified as BI-RADS 5 (**Fig. 5.1c, d**).

Ultrasonography

Hypoechoic mass with ill-defined margins in the left breast, measuring 20 × 11 × 12 mm. Classified as BI-RADS 5. The lesion definitely correlates with clinical and mammographic findings (**Fig. 5.1e, f**).

Further Case History

Ultrasound-guided core-needle biopsy was performed, identifying the lesion as grade 2 invasive carcinoma (no special type).

Final Diagnosis

Invasive breast carcinoma.

Discussion

The spiculated mass is defined much more clearly on three-dimensional (3D) tomosynthesis than on standard mammograms. In this case, tomosynthesis aids in mass detection and localization, but it does not increase sensitivity or specificity because the lesion was also visible on mammograms.

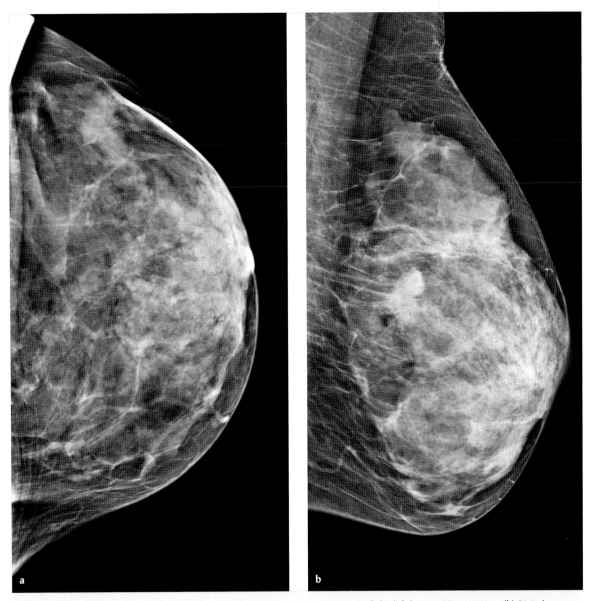

Fig. 5.1 Case 1. 72-year-old woman with skin retraction. **(a)** Digital mammogram of the left breast, CC projection. **(b)** Digital mammogram of the left breast, MLO projection.

continued ▶

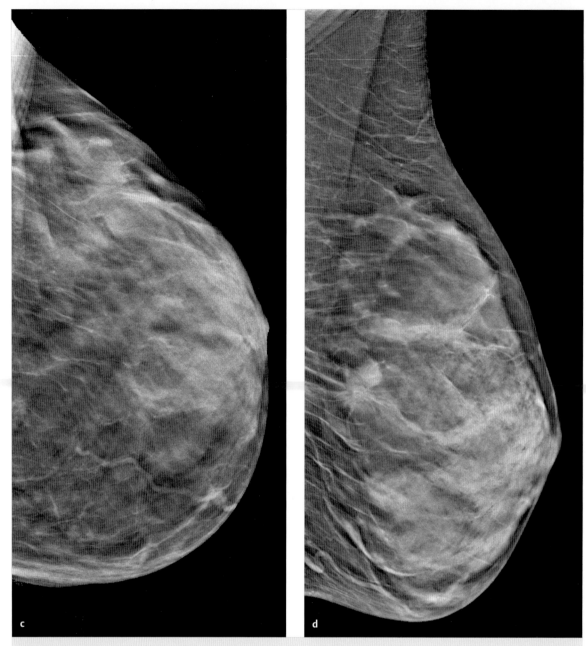

Fig. 5.1 (continued) Case 1. 72-year-old woman with skin retraction. **(c)** Single slice from 3D tomosynthesis data set of the left breast, CC projection. **(d)** Single slice from 3D tomosynthesis data set of the left breast, MLO projection.

continued ▶

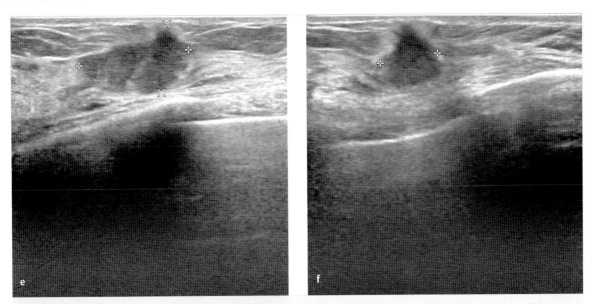

Fig. 5.1 (continued) Case 1. 72-year-old woman with skin retraction. **(e)** Ultrasound scan of the mass. **(f)** Ultrasound scan of the mass, second plane.

5.2.2 Case 2

History

Woman 41 years of age with no family history of breast cancer, not on hormone therapy. She is a primipara (P1) and breastfed for 8 months. Status post-excisional biopsy of the left breast in 2008 with benign histology.

Mammography

Left breast: ACR 4. Spiculated lesion visible in the MLO view, less visible in the CC view but presumably located in the upper outer quadrant. Classified as BI-RADS 4 (**Fig. 5.2a, b**).

DBT

DBT of the left breast in the MLO projection. A lead bead has been placed to mark the suspicious area. DBT displays the spiculated lesion with much greater clarity than mammography (**Fig. 5.2c**, **Video 5.1**).

Ultrasonography

Prepectoral hypoechoic area with ill-defined margins in the upper outer quadrant of the left breast, measuring $1.0 \times 1.1 \times 1.0$ cm (**Fig. 5.2d**).

Further Case History

Ultrasound-guided core-needle biopsy revealed fibrocystic changes. As this did not adequately explain the spiculated mass, stereotactic vacuum biopsy was performed. Histology showed fibrocystic changes, marked hyalinosis, and periductal fibrosis. This finding was interpreted as a radial scar and classified as a B3 lesion. Local excision was performed after stereotactic wire localization.

Final Diagnosis

Radial scar.

Discussion

This case illustrates the superiority of DBT in the detection of spiculated lesions. After the site has been marked with a lead bead, DBT can establish definite correlation of the sonographic and mammographic findings.

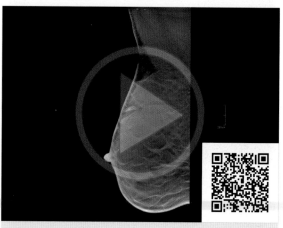

Video 5.1 Case 2. DBT data set, MLO projection with a lead bead marker. Spiculated mass.

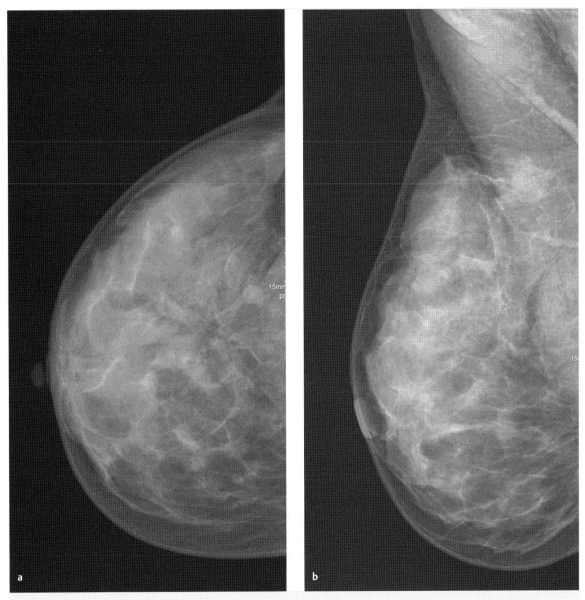

Fig. 5.2 Case 2. 41-year-old woman, status post-excisional biopsy with benign histology. **(a)** Mammogram in the CC projection. **(b)** Mammogram in the MLO projection.

continued ▶

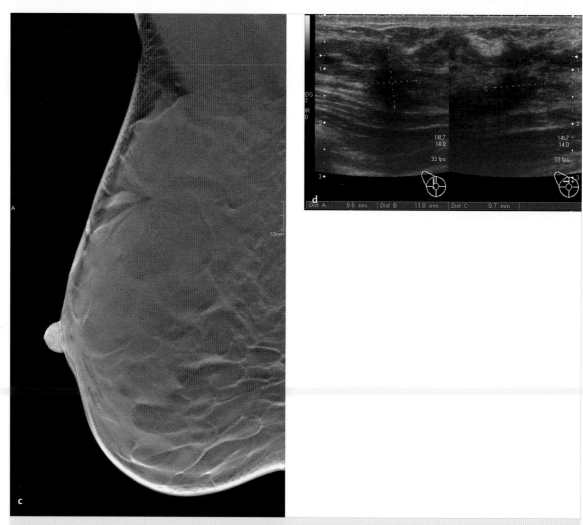

Fig. 5.2 (continued) Case 2. 41-year-old woman, status post-excisional biopsy with benign histology. **(c)** Representative tomosynthesis slice, MLO projection. **(d)** Ultrasound scans of the lesion.

5.2.3 Case 3

History

Asymptomatic 60-year-old woman with a family history of breast cancer, 9 years after excisional biopsy of the left breast for atypical ductal hyperplasia.

Mammography

Right breast: ACR 3. Moderately coarse pattern of fibrocystic changes. CC projection shows a 5-mm area of slightly increased retroareolar density approximately 3 cm from the nipple (**Fig. 5.3a**), not visible in the oblique view (**Fig. 5.3b**). Classified as BI-RADS 4.

DBT

CC and MLO tomosynthesis views of the right breast demonstrate a spiculated mass located approximately 3 cm behind the nipple. Classified as BI-RADS 5 (**Fig. 5.3c, d**).

Ultrasonography

Hypoechoic mass with ill-defined margins in the right breast, measuring $6 \times 3 \times 3$ mm, consisting of two parts. The lesion correlates with the mammographic findings. Classified as BI-RADS 5. (**Fig. 5.3e, f**).

Further Case History

Ultrasound-guided core-needle biopsy of the right breast identified the lesion histologically as a 7-mm grade 2 carcinoma of the invasive lobular type.

Final Diagnosis

Invasive lobular carcinoma.

Discussion

Only one mammographic view shows an area of increased density, while tomosynthesis clearly demonstrates a spiculated mass. In this case, then, tomosynthesis provides better lesion detection and characterization than mammography.

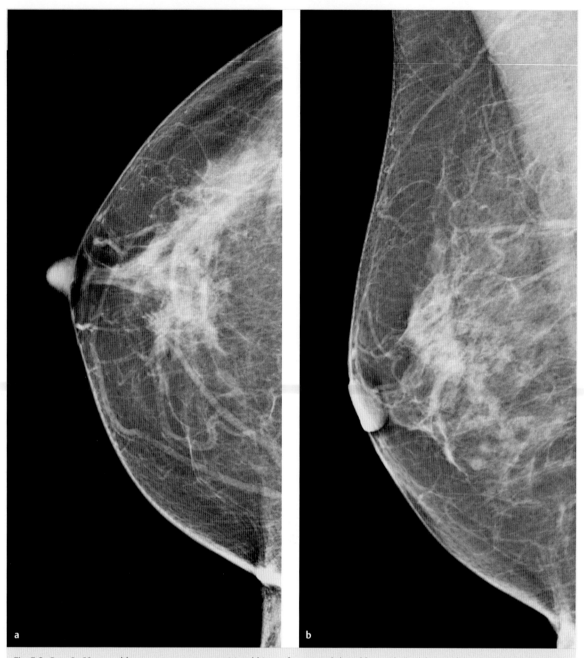

Fig. 5.3 Case 3. 60-year-old woman, status post-excisional biopsy for atypical ductal hyperplasia. **(a)** Digital mammogram of the right breast, CC projection. **(b)** Digital mammogram of the right breast, MLO projection.

continued ▶

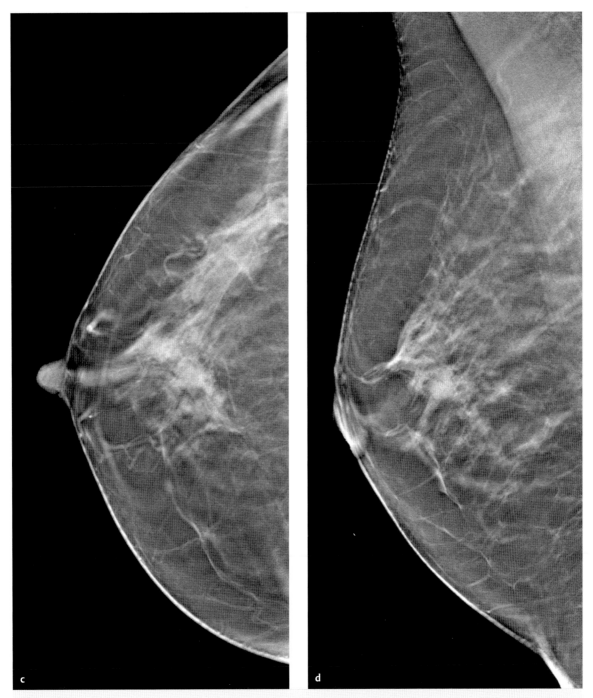

c

d

Fig. 5.3 (continued) Case 3. 60-year-old woman, status post-excisional biopsy for atypical ductal hyperplasia. **(c)** Single slice from 3D tomosynthesis data set of the right breast, CC projection. **(d)** Single slice from 3D tomosynthesis data set of the right breast, MLO projection.

continued ▶

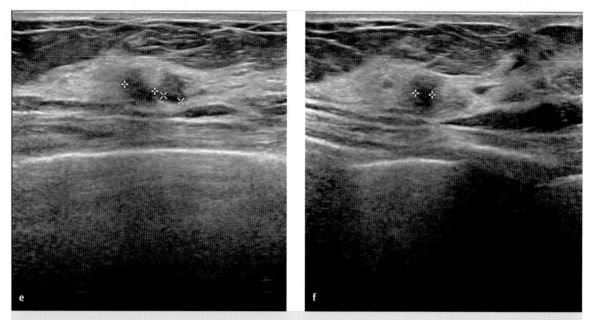

Fig. 5.3 (continued) Case 3. 60-year-old woman, status post-excisional biopsy for atypical ductal hyperplasia. **(e)** Ultrasound scan of the mass. **(f)** Ultrasound scan of the mass, second plane.

5.2.4 Case 4

History

Woman 44 years of age with no family history of breast cancer, not on hormone therapy. She is a primigravida (G1), P1, and breastfed for 6 months.

Mammography

Right breast: ACR 2. Spiculated mass in the upper outer quadrant, classified as BI-RADS 4 (**Fig. 5.4a, c**). Additional suspected intramammary lymph node. Left breast: ACR 2. Classified as BI-RADS 2 (**Fig. 5.4b, d**).

DBT

CC view shows a spiculated mass in the upper outer quadrant of the right breast (**Fig. 5.4e**) and an intramammary lymph node (**Fig. 5.4f, Video 5.2**).

Ultrasonography

Ultrasonography does not show a correlate for the mammographic lesion.

Further Case History

The mass was investigated by stereotactic core-needle biopsy.

Final Diagnosis

Moderately differentiated carcinoma (no special type) with associated ductal carcinoma in situ (DCIS).

Discussion

Both the benign and malignant breast lesions can be accurately detected and characterized by tomosynthesis.

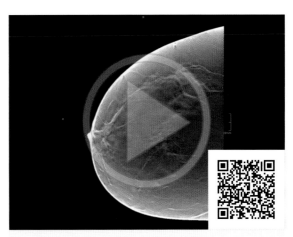

Video 5.2 Case 4. DBT data set of the right breast, CC projection. Spiculated mass and intramammary lymph node.

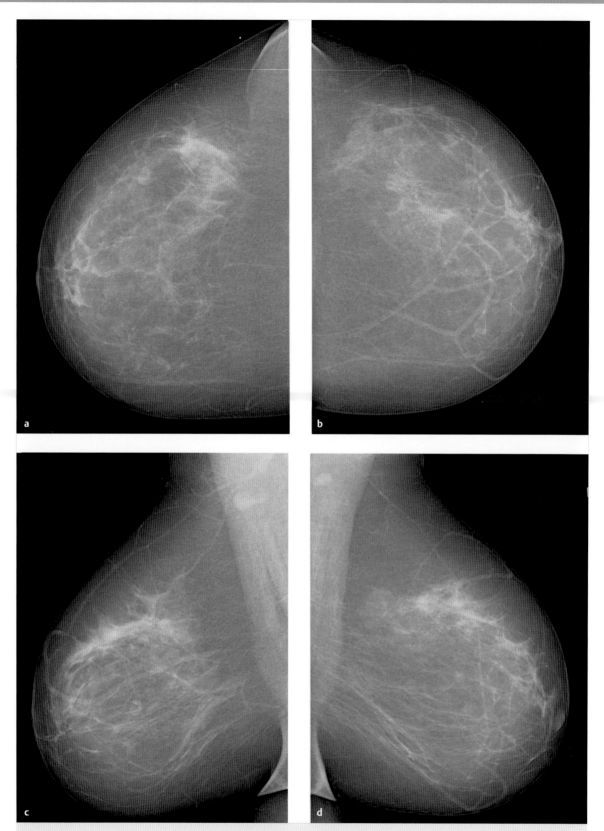

Fig. 5.4 Case 4. Screening examination of a 44-year-old woman. **(a)** Digital mammogram of the right breast, CC projection. ACR 2. Spiculated mass in the upper outer quadrant. Suspected intramammary lymph node. **(b)** Digital mammogram of the left breast, CC projection. **(c)** Digital mammogram of the right breast, MLO projection. **(d)** Digital mammogram of the left breast, MLO projection.

continued ▶

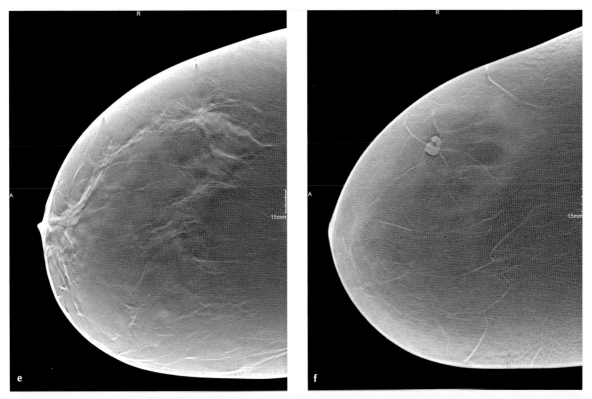

Fig. 5.4 (continued) Case 4. Screening examination of a 44-year-old woman. (**e**) DBT of the right breast, CC projection. (**f**) DBT of the right breast, CC projection.

5.2.5 Case 5

History

Follow-up of an asymptomatic 78-year-old woman 7 years after diagnosis of DCIS. She has a known, firm, only slightly mobile 1.5-cm mass at the 2 o'clock position in the left breast. The mass is located 6 cm from the nipple, within a scarred area. No other clinical abnormalities.

Mammography

Left breast: ACR 2. Architectural distortion is present in the upper outer quadrant, owing to scarring. A 1.8-cm lucency with smooth margins and shell-like calcifications is visible in the scarred area. The mammographic architectural distortion correlates with the palpable mass and represents known liponecrosis. Vascular calcification is also noted. BI-RADS 2 (**Fig. 5.5a, b**).

DBT

DBT of the left breast in the MLO projection. A scarred area after segmental mastectomy appears as an architectural distortion. The scarred region contains a typically well-circumscribed area of liponecrosis with central lucency and shell-like calcifications. Vascular calcification is also found. Classified as BI-RADS 2 (**Fig. 5.5c, d**).

Final Diagnosis

Liponecrosis at the segmental mastectomy site.

Discussion

Tomosynthesis provides excellent delineation of the liponecrosis (oil cyst) in the scarred area. The 3D technique provides views that are not obscured by superimposed tissues.

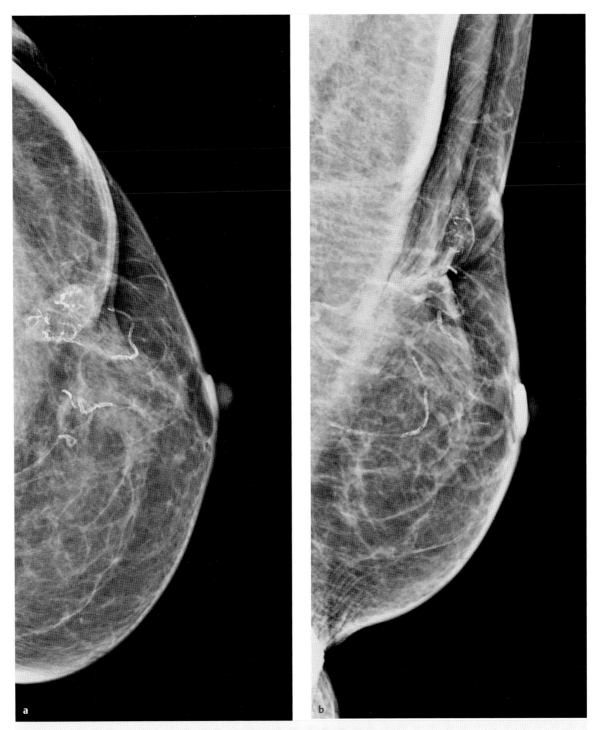

Fig. 5.5 Case 5. Follow-up imaging of a 78-year-old woman with a history of DCIS. **(a)** Digital mammogram of the left breast, CC projection. **(b)** Digital mammogram of the left breast, MLO projection.

continued ▶

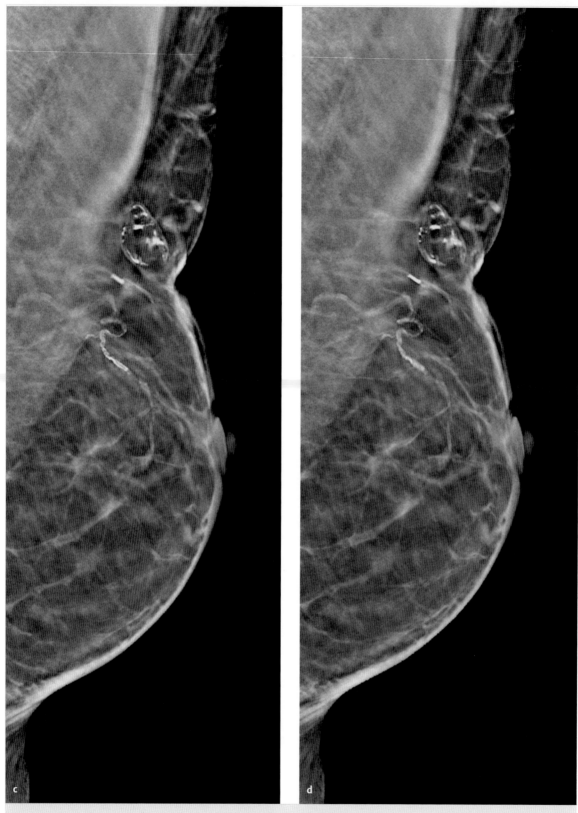

Fig. 5.5 (continued) Case 5. Follow-up imaging of a 78-year-old woman with a history of DCIS. **(c)** Single slice from 3D tomosynthesis data set of the left breast, MLO projection. **(d)** Single slice from 3D tomosynthesis data set of the left breast, MLO projection.

5.2.6 Case 6

History

Asymptomatic 71-year-old woman with no visible or palpable abnormalities in either breast. Status post-ovarian cancer 10 years earlier.

Mammography

Right breast: ACR 3. Nodular pattern of fibrocystic changes. A 5-mm prepectoral mass is visible in the upper outer quadrant at the 11 o'clock position, 5 cm from the nipple, and has partially irregular margins. Classified as BI-RADS 4 (**Fig. 5.6a, b**).

DBT

MLO view of the right breast shows an elliptical mass with smooth margins and central lucency, typical of a nonspecific lymph node. Right breast is reclassified as BI-RADS 2 (**Fig. 5.6c**).

Final Diagnosis

Nonspecific right intramammary lymph node.

Discussion

The mass is clearly visualized by supplemental 3D tomosynthesis. DBT improves specificity in this case and permits downgrading of the BI-RADS 4 mammographic lesion to BI-RADS 2.

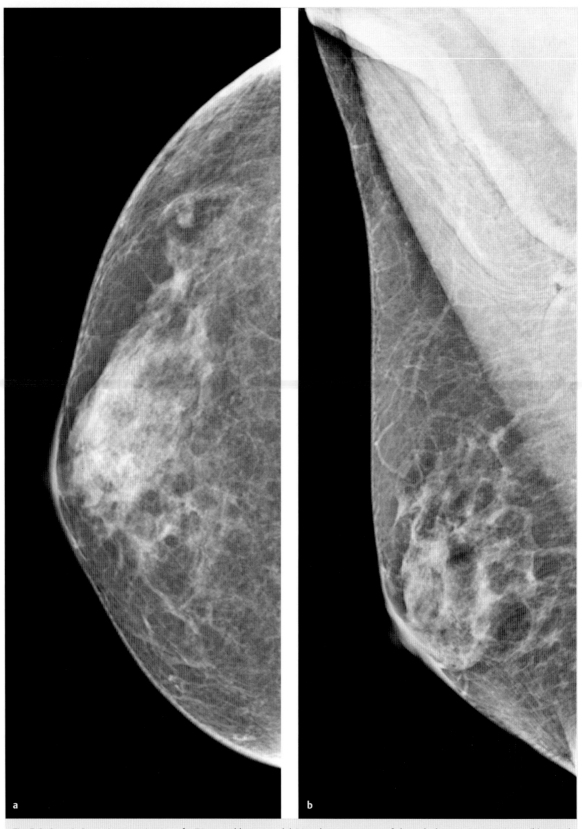

Fig. 5.6 Case 6. Screening examination of a 71-year-old woman. **(a)** Digital mammogram of the right breast, CC projection. **(b)** Digital mammogram of the right breast, MLO projection.

continued ▶

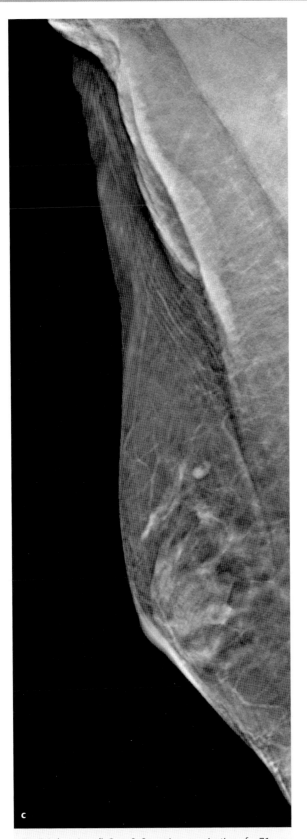

c

Fig. 5.6 (continued) Case 6. Screening examination of a 71-year-old woman. **(c)** Single slice from 3D tomosynthesis data set of the right breast, MLO projection.

5.2.7 Case 7

History

Asymptomatic 51-year-old woman. G1, P1, did not breastfeed. She has an older sister diagnosed with breast cancer at age 50 years. Patient is not on hormone therapy.

Mammography

Right breast: ACR 3. No mass or microcalcifications. Classified as BI-RADS 2 (**Fig. 5.7a, c**). Left breast: ACR 3. Central, questionable spiculated lesion in the CC view with no visible correlate in the MLO view. Classified as BI-RADS 4 (**Fig. 5.7b, d**).

DBT

Tomosynthesis shows a definite spiculated lesion in the upper central breast (**Fig. 5.7e**, **Video 5.3**).

Ultrasonography

Hypoechoic mass with ill-defined margins in the upper breast, 1.3 × 0.9 × 0.4 cm (**Fig. 5.7f**).

Further Case History

Ultrasound-guided core-needle biopsy identified the mass as moderately differentiated invasive lobular carcinoma, which was marked with a clip after the intervention. Final diagnosis after segmental mastectomy: 1.8-cm invasive lobular carcinoma accompanied by foci of atypical lobular hyperplasia.

Final Diagnosis

Invasive lobular carcinoma.

Discussion

The mammograms were interpreted externally by two experienced readers. One scored the images as BI-RADS 2, the other as BI-RADS 4. This prompted a recall for further evaluation. The spiculated lesion can be detected more easily and confidently on tomosynthesis than on mammography. In this case, however, breast ultrasonography would also have been sufficient to confirm the diagnosis.

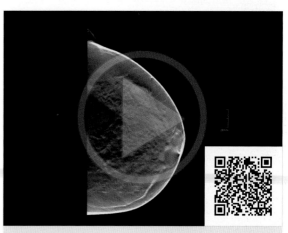

Video 5.3 Case 7. DBT data set of the left breast, CC projection. Spiculated lesion in the upper central portion of the breast.

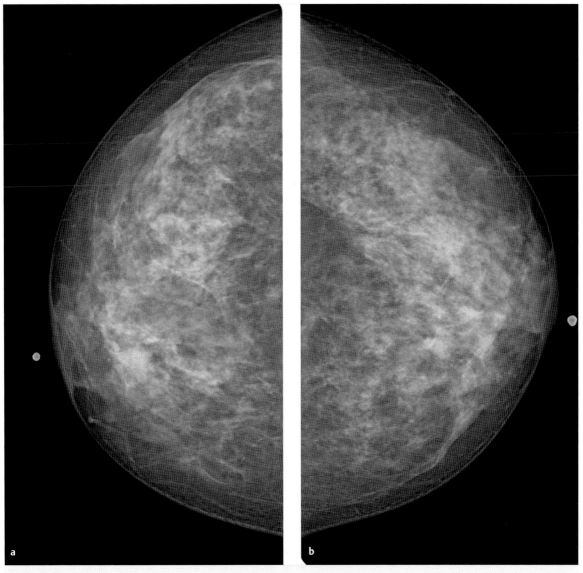

Fig. 5.7 Case 7. Screening examination of a 51-year-old woman. **(a)** Digital mammogram of the right breast, CC projection. **(b)** Digital mammogram of the left breast, CC projection.

continued ▶

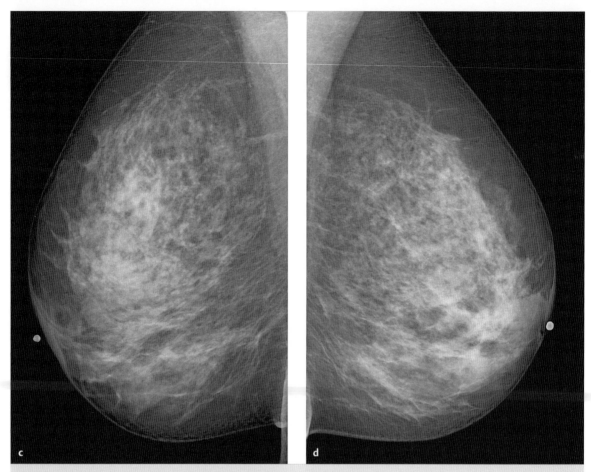

Fig. 5.7 (continued) Case 7. Screening examination of a 51-year-old woman. **(c)** Digital mammogram of the right breast, MLO projection. **(d)** Digital mammogram of the left breast, MLO projection.

continued ▶

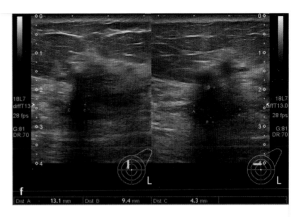

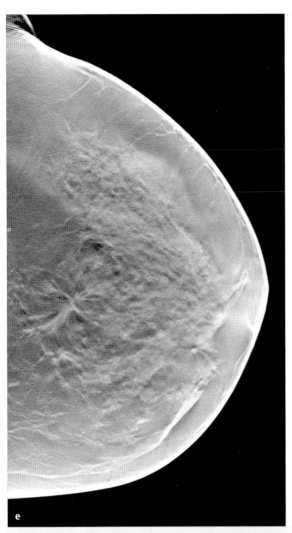

Fig. 5.7 (continued) Case 7. Screening examination of a 51-year-old woman. **(e)** Single slice from 3D tomosynthesis data set of the left breast, CC projection. **(f)** Ultrasound scans of the mass.

5.2.8 Case 8

History

Asymptomatic woman with three children, each breastfed for 3 months. She has no family history of breast cancer and is on transdermal hormone replacement therapy (HRT). No palpable masses or enlarged locoregional lymph nodes. Well-healed scars are present from previous bilateral open breast biopsies (2000).

Mammography

Right breast: ACR 3. Skin and nipple appear normal. No suspicious mammographic masses or suspicious microcalcifications. Classified as BI-RADS 1 (**Fig. 5.8a**, **c**). Left breast: ACR 3. Skin and nipple appear normal. CC projection shows an 8-mm mass in the medial half of the left breast, 4 cm from the nipple. No visible correlate in the MLO projection. No suspicious microcalcifications. Classified as BI-RADS 4 (**Fig. 5.8b**, **d**).

Ultrasonography

Targeted ultrasound scans of the left breast show a mass in the lower inner quadrant, measuring 6.6 × 5.2 × 7.6 mm, with central internal echoes and no architectural distortion (**Fig. 5.8e**). Lesion location was marked on the skin with a lead bead marker.

DBT

DBT of the left breast with the skin marker in place. CC view demonstrates an elongated, low-density mass with predominantly smooth margins located close to the marker (**Fig. 5.8f**). A similar mass is found at a more cranial level in the same region (**Fig. 5.8g**). The images suggest a low index of suspicion. Classified as BI-RADS 3 (**Video 5.4**).

Further Case History

Based on the suspicious mammographic mass and its ultrasonographic correlate, detailed informed consent was obtained for an ultrasound-guided core-needle biopsy of the left breast. Histology revealed adenosis, ordinary ductal hyperplasia, columnar cell metaplasia, and focal oncocytic metaplasia, with no evidence of malignancy (B2). The findings were unchanged at 1-year follow-up.

Final Diagnosis

Fibrocystic changes with no evidence of malignancy.

Discussion

The suspicious mammographic mass was identified as a summation artifact on tomosynthesis, but the patient still wanted a definitive histologic diagnosis. In retrospect, and based on growing experience with tomosynthesis, biopsy could have been withheld in the present case.

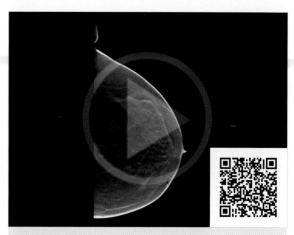

Video 5.4 Case 8. DBT data set of the left breast, CC projection with a lead bead marker. Two well-circumscribed, elongated low-density lesions.

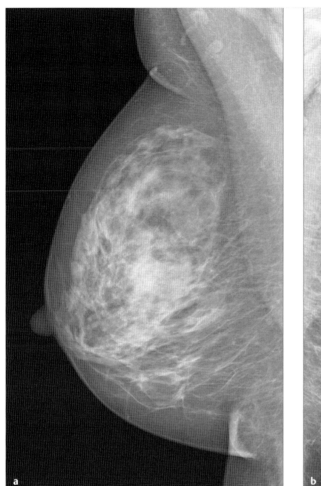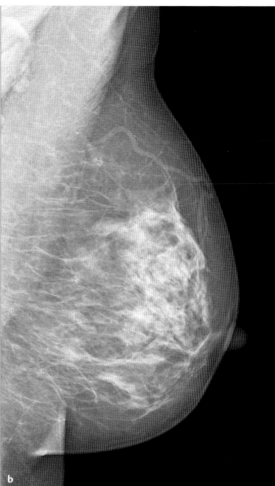

Fig. 5.8 Case 8. Asymptomatic patient had previous bilateral open biopsies with benign results. **(a)** Digital mammogram of the right breast, MLO projection. **(b)** Digital mammogram of the left breast, MLO projection.

continued ▶

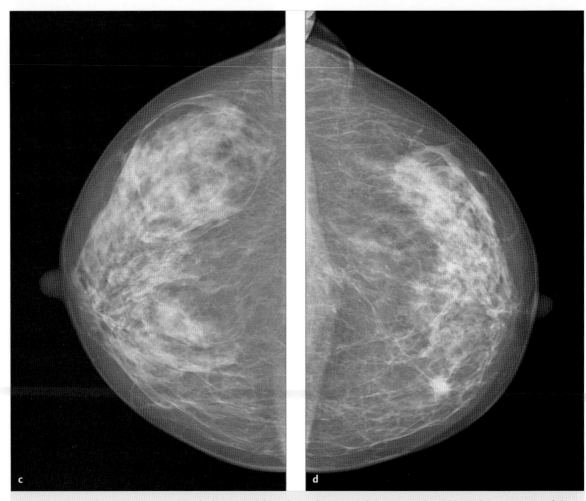

Fig. 5.8 (continued) Asymptomatic patient had previous bilateral open biopsies with benign results. **(c)** Digital mammogram of the right breast, CC projection. **(d)** Digital mammogram of the left breast, CC projection.

continued ▶

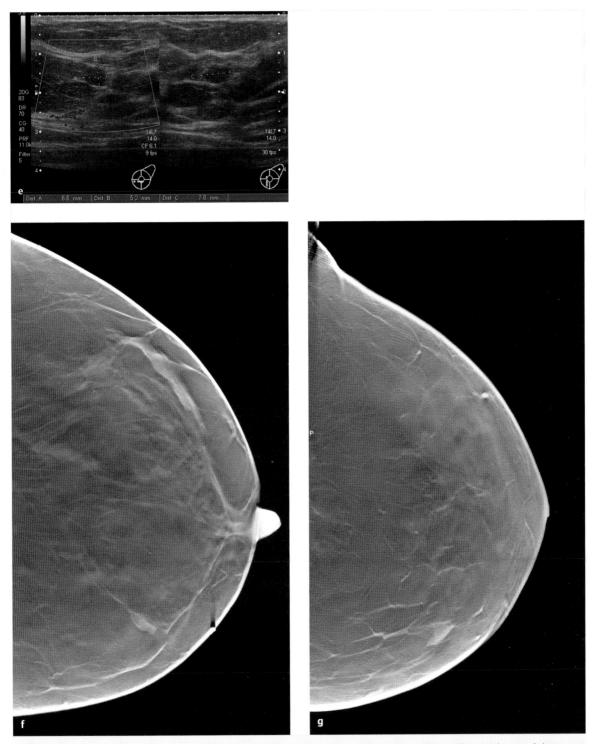

Fig. 5.8 (continued) Asymptomatic patient had previous bilateral open biopsies with benign results. **(e)** Ultrasound scans of the mass. **(f)** Single slice from 3D tomosynthesis data set of the left breast, CC projection. **(g)** Single slice from 3D tomosynthesis data set of the left breast, CC projection.

5.2.9 Case 9

History

Asymptomatic 74-year-old woman. G2, P1, breastfed for 6 months. No family history of breast cancer, no hormone therapy. No palpable masses. The right breast has been smaller than the left for many years. Right nipple retraction has been present for approximately 6 months.

Mammography

Right breast: ACR 2. CC view shows a spiculated lesion in the outer half of the breast and a retroareolar density with architectural distortion. Classified as BI-RADS 4 (**Fig. 5.9a, c**). Left breast: ACR 2. No focal lesions. Classified as BI-RADS 2 (**Fig. 5.9b, d**).

DBT

DBT of the right breast in the CC projection. The mammographic lesion in the lower outer quadrant appears on tomosynthesis as an ill-defined mass with radiating spicules (**Fig. 5.9e**). DBT also shows an ill-defined retroareolar density measuring up to 1.5 cm in its largest dimension (**Fig. 5.9f**). Overall classification is BI-RADS 5 (**Video 5.5**).

Ultrasonography

Scans of the right breast show a hypoechoic retroareolar mass with irregular margins, measuring 1.1 × 1.1 × 1.1 cm (**Fig. 5.9g**). Ultrasonography does not detect a mass at the site of the other mammographic density.

Further Case History

Ultrasound-guided core-needle biopsy of the retroareolar mass in the right breast showed moderately differentiated invasive carcinoma of no special type (NST), with a small intraductal component. Classified histologically as a B5 b lesion. The mass in the lower outer quadrant was also biopsied after wire localization and proved to be a moderately differentiated invasive lobular carcinoma.

Final Diagnosis

Moderately differentiated invasive carcinoma NST in the retroareolar area of the right breast, plus moderately differentiated invasive lobular carcinoma in the lower outer quadrant.

Discussion

The retroareolar lesion is best demonstrated by ultrasonography, while the lesion in the lower outer quadrant is most accurately detected and characterized by tomosynthesis. This case illustrates the value of breast ultrasonography and tomosynthesis as complementary modalities.

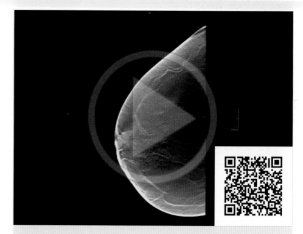

Video 5.5 Case 9. DBT data set of the right breast, CC projection. Ill-defined lesion with radiating spicules in the lower outer quadrant of the breast, plus an ill-defined retroareolar density up to 1.5 cm in its largest dimension.

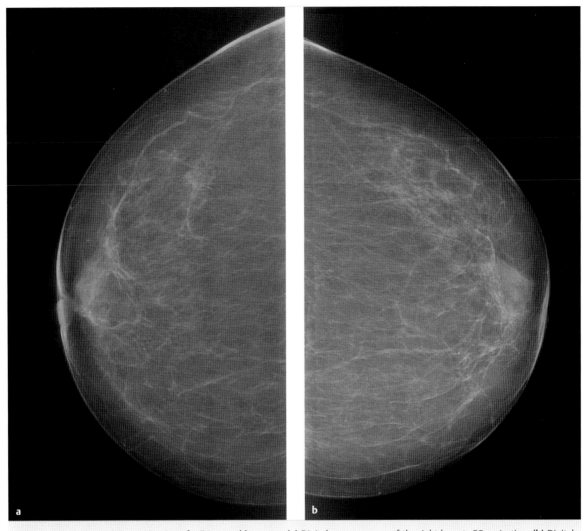

Fig. 5.9 Case 9. Screening examination of a 74-year-old woman. **(a)** Digital mammogram of the right breast, CC projection. **(b)** Digital mammogram of the left breast, CC projection.

continued ▶

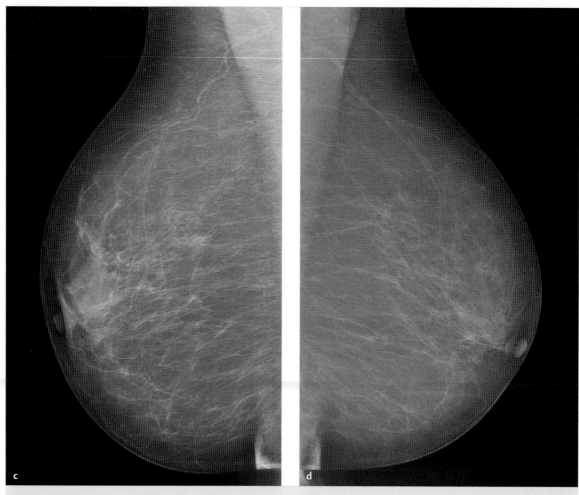

Fig. 5.9 (continued) Case 9. Screening examination of a 74-year-old woman. **(c)** Digital mammogram of the right breast, MLO projection. **(d)** Digital mammogram of the left breast, MLO projection.

continued ▶

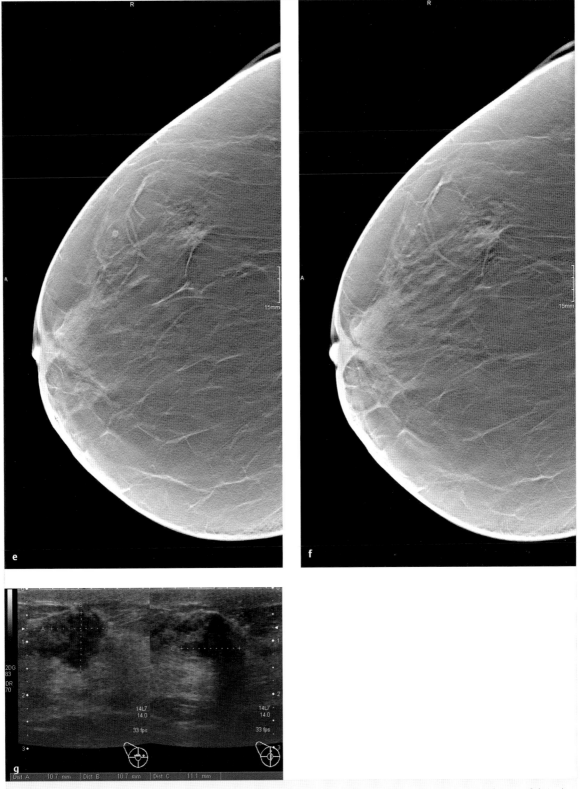

Fig. 5.9 (continued) Case 9. Screening examination of a 74-year-old woman. **(e)** Single slice from 3D tomosynthesis data set of the right breast, CC projection. **(f)** Single slice from 3D tomosynthesis data set of the right breast, CC projection. **(g)** Ultrasound scans of the mass.

5.2.10 Case 10

History

A 42-year-old woman with significant bilateral fibrocystic breast changes and right mastodynia. No family history of breast cancer. No visible abnormalities. Palpable findings are consistent with fibrocystic changes.

Mammography

Bilateral mammograms in the CC projection. Both breasts are classified as ACR 4. Images show a fibrocystic parenchymal pattern with increased radiographic density. No masses or microcalcifications are seen. Both breasts are classified as BI-RADS 2 (**Fig. 5.10a, b**).

DBT

Bilateral DBT in the MLO projection. Tomosynthesis also shows significant bilateral fibrocystic changes with increased parenchymal density. Both breasts are classified as BI-RADS 2 (**Fig. 5.10c–f**).

Ultrasonography

No suspicious masses in either breast.

Final Diagnosis

Significant bilateral fibrocystic changes. BI-RADS 2.

Discussion

In this patient with very dense breast parenchyma, only one mammographic view was obtained (CC) and this was supplemented by tomosynthesis in the MLO projection. With this combination, which has been investigated in several studies, mammography can detect microcalcifications, while complementary-view tomosynthesis can detect or exclude masses. Ultrasonography is also a necessary adjunct, however, even when tomosynthesis is used.

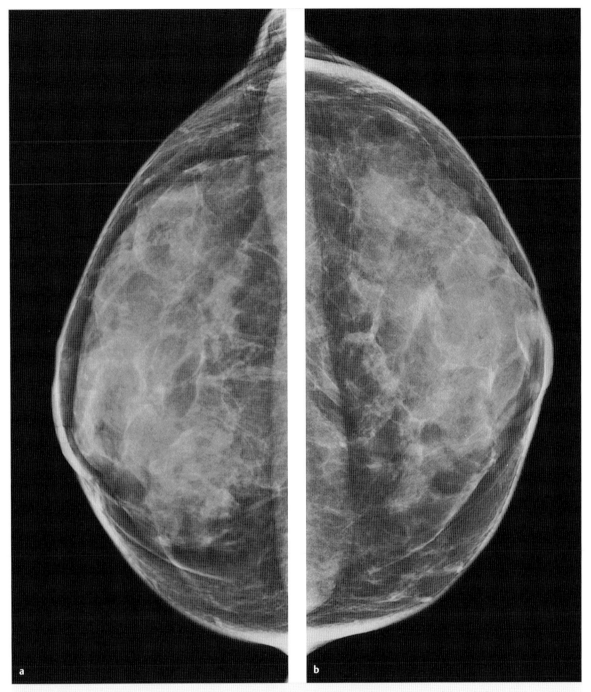

Fig. 5.10 Case 10. Significant fibrocystic changes in a 42-year-old woman. (a) Digital mammogram of the right breast, CC projection. (b) Digital mammogram of the left breast, CC projection.

continued ▶

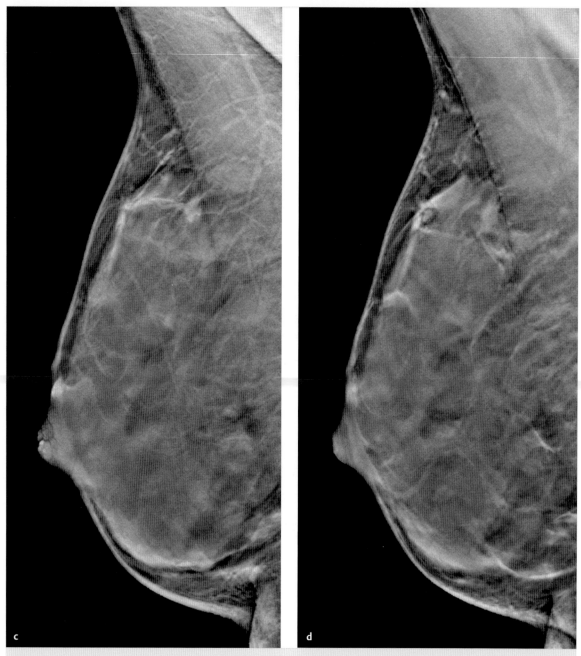

Fig. 5.10 (continued) Case 10. Significant fibrocystic changes in a 42-year-old woman. **(c)** Single slice from 3D tomosynthesis data set of the right breast, MLO projection. **(d)** Single slice from 3D tomosynthesis data set of the right breast, MLO projection.

continued ▶

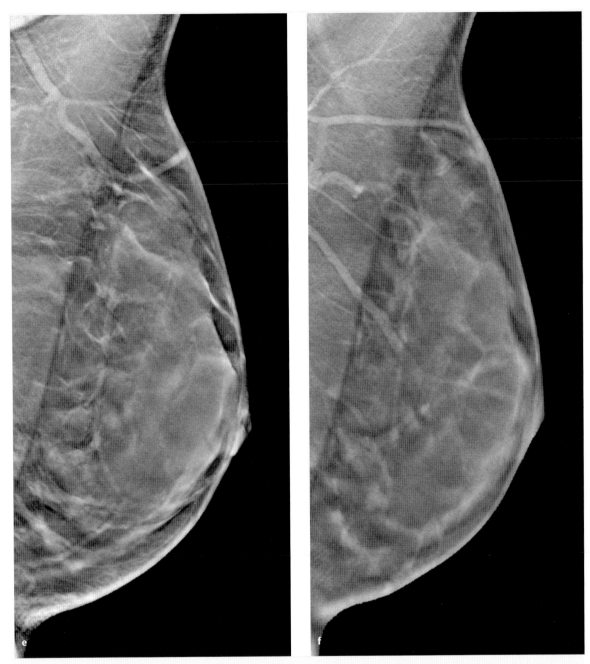

Fig. 5.10 (continued) Case 10. Significant fibrocystic changes in a 42-year-old woman. **(e)** Single slice from 3D tomosynthesis data set of the left breast, MLO projection. **(f)** Single slice from 3D tomosynthesis data set of the left breast, MLO projection.

5.2.11 Case 11

History

A 42-year-old woman found three palpable masses in the periareolar region during breast self-examination. Clinical examination finds corresponding firm masses up to 1 cm in size, suspicious for malignancy, in the periareolar region of the right breast. They are located at the 5 o'clock, 9 o'clock, and 11 o'clock positions.

Mammography

Right breast: ACR 4. Patchy fibrocystic changes with no evidence of masses or microcalcifications. Right breast changes are classified as BI-RADS 2 (**Fig. 5.11a, b**).

DBT

DBT of the right breast in the MLO projection. Supplemental tomosynthesis of the right breast shows no abnormalities at the location of the palpable masses. Classified as BI-RADS 2 (**Fig. 5.11c, d**).

Breast Magnetic Resonance Imagining (MRI)

MRI of the right breast demonstrates the three periareolar lesions as spiculated masses with suspicious enhancement and rapid washout (**Fig. 5.11e**).

Ultrasonography

On ultrasound scans of the right breast, the three suspicious palpable masses appear as hypoechoic lesions with ill-defined margins that coincide precisely with the clinical findings. Classified as BI-RADS 5 (**Fig. 5.11f, g**).

Further Case History

The three masses were investigated by ultrasound-guided core-needle biopsy, which identified each lesion as grade 2 invasive carcinoma NST. Their individual sizes were determined histologically as 7, 8, and 11 mm.

Final Diagnosis

Multifocal invasive carcinoma NST.

Discussion

Ultrasonography and MRI are the only modalities that showed abnormalities at the sites of the three palpable masses. Owing to the high radiographic density of the breast parenchyma (ACR 4), neither mammography nor tomosynthesis could detect the lesions in this patient. Both techniques were false negative because even in DBT, lesion detection requires a density difference between the tumor and surrounding tissue. Tomosynthesis cannot exclude tumors in dense glandular tissue, and an accurate diagnosis in these cases always requires additional evaluation by ultrasonography.

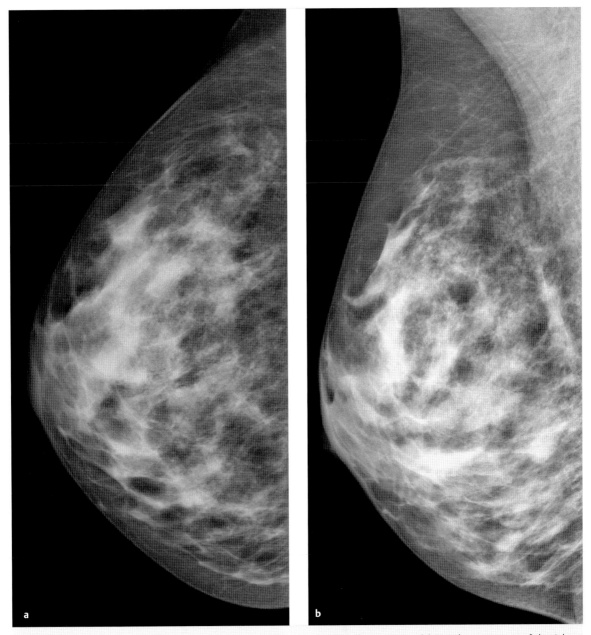

Fig. 5.11 Case 11. 42-year-old woman with palpable masses found on breast self-examination. **(a)** Digital mammogram of the right breast, CC projection. **(b)** Digital mammogram of the right breast, MLO projection.

continued ▶

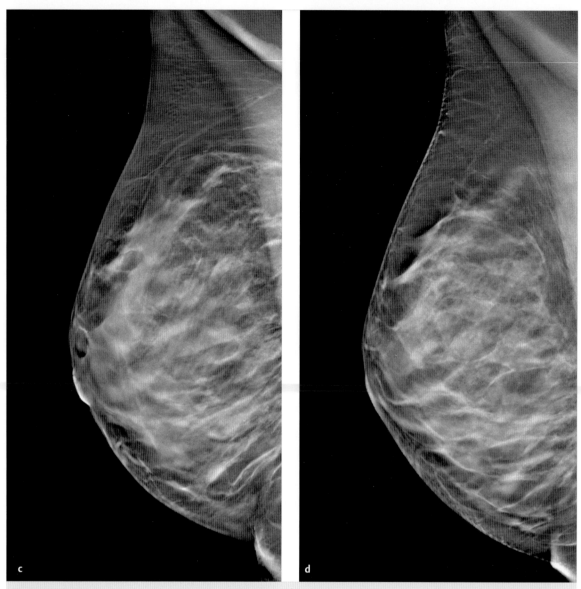

Fig. 5.11 (continued) Case 11. 42-year-old woman with palpable masses found on breast self-examination. **(c)** Single slice from 3D tomosynthesis data set of the right breast, MLO projection. **(d)** Single slice from 3D tomosynthesis data set of the right breast, MLO projection.

continued ▶

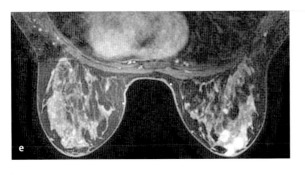

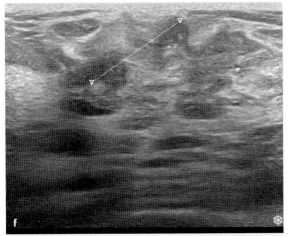

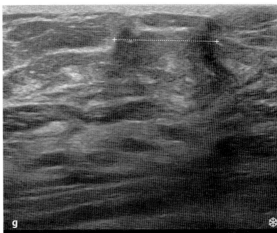

Fig. 5.11 (continued) Case 11. 42-year-old woman with palpable masses found on breast self-examination. **(e)** MRI of the right breast: axial T 1-weighted sequence after contrast administration. **(f)** Ultrasound scan of the masses (12.5-MHz probe). **(g)** Ultrasound scan of the masses, second plane.

5.2.12 Case 12

History

Asymptomatic 71-year-old woman. G1, P1, breastfed for several weeks. Patient is on HRT. No family history of breast cancer. Localized firmness of the right breast is noted at the 9 o'clock position, with associated skin retraction when the arm is raised.

Mammography

Right breast: ACR 3. MLO projection shows areas of lipoid necrosis plus architectural distortion in the upper outer quadrant. CC projection shows asymmetry but no definite correlate with the MLO findings. Classified as BI-RADS 4 (**Fig. 5.12a, c**). Left breast: ACR 3. No mammographic lesions. Multiple sites of lipoid necrosis. Classified as BI-RADS 2 (**Fig. 5.12b, d**).

DBT

MLO view of the right breast confirms the architectural distortion, which is best appreciated by scrolling through the complete DBT data set. Classified as BI-RADS 4 (**Fig. 5.12e, Video 5.6**).

Ultrasonography

Ultrasound scans of the right breast demonstrate an irregular hypoechoic mass with ill-defined margins at the 9 o'clock position, measuring 0.9 × 2.2 × 1.6 cm. Suspected tumor spicules radiate to the skin (**Fig. 5.12f**).

Further Case History

Ultrasound-guided core-needle biopsy identified the mass as poorly differentiated invasive carcinoma. Treatment consisted of breast-conserving surgery and adjuvant radiotherapy.

Final Diagnosis

Poorly differentiated carcinoma NST 3 cm in diameter.

Discussion

The architectural distortion in this case is particularly well demonstrated by scrolling through the tomosynthesis data set. Ultrasonography is best for tumor detection. All the modalities underestimated tumor size relative to actual histologic size.

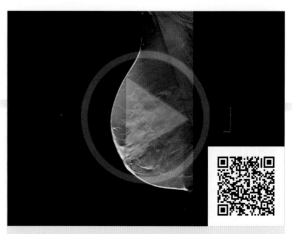

Video 5.6 Case 12. DBT data set of the right breast, MLO projection. Architectural distortion.

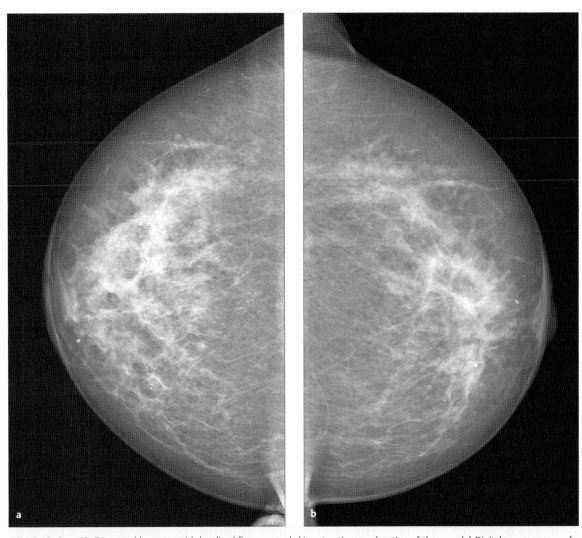

Fig. 5.12 Case 12. 71-year-old woman with localized firmness and skin retraction on elevation of the arm. **(a)** Digital mammogram of the right breast, CC projection. **(b)** Digital mammogram of the left breast, CC projection.

continued ▶

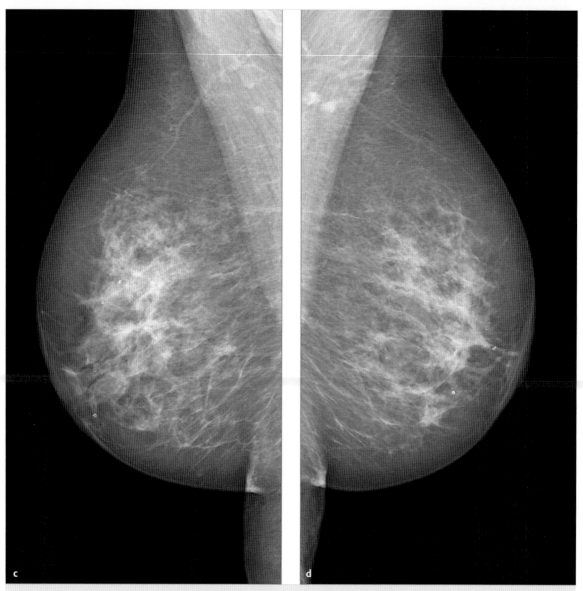

Fig. 5.12 (continued) Case 12. 71-year-old woman with localized firmness and skin retraction on elevation of the arm. **(c)** Digital mammogram of the right breast, MLO projection. **(d)** Digital mammogram of the left breast, MLO projection.

continued ▶

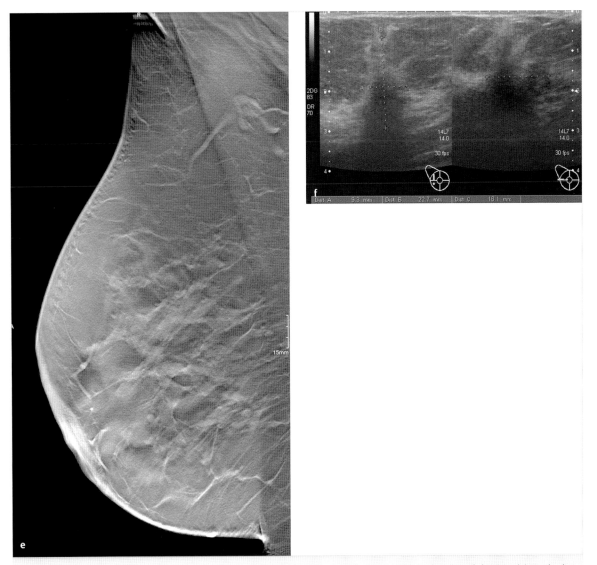

Fig. 5.12 (continued) Case 12. 71-year-old woman with localized firmness and skin retraction on elevation of the arm. **(e)** Single slice from 3D tomosynthesis data set of the right breast, MLO projection. **(f)** Ultrasound scans of the mass.

5.2.13 Case 13

History

A 59-year-old woman has a family history of breast cancer and known fibrocystic changes. She has no complaints and no visible or palpable abnormalities in either breast.

Mammography

Left breast: ACR 3. A mass measuring 8 × 9 mm, partially obscured by parenchyma but elsewhere showing relatively smooth margins, is located approximately 5 cm from the nipple at the 11 o'clock position. A second, smaller mass of similar shape, 4 mm in diameter, is located 6 cm from the nipple at the 1 o'clock position. Both lesions are classified mammographically as BI-RADS 4 (**Fig. 5.13a, b**).

DBT

DBT of the left breast in the MLO projection. Both masses have completely smooth margins by tomosynthesis and are downgraded to BI-RADS 2 (**Fig. 5.13c**).

Ultrasonography

Ultrasound scans of the left breast show two well-circumscribed, elliptical, echo-free masses at the 11 o'clock and 1 o'clock positions. The lesion at the 11 o'clock position measures 9 × 8 mm and shows posterior echo enhancement (**Fig. 5.13d, e**). The lesion at the 1 o'clock position measures 3 × 4 mm (**Fig. 5.13f, g**). Classified as BI-RADS 2.

Final Diagnosis

BI-RADS 2, benign breast cysts.

Discussion

Tomosynthesis allows a more precise characterization of focal lesions than mammography because the margins are not obscured by superimposed parenchyma. Several large studies have confirmed that tomosynthesis can lower recall rates in screening.

Ultrasonography in the present case confirms the tomosynthesis findings and is unquestionably the preferred technique for evaluating breast cysts. Compared with the combination of mammography and ultrasonography, tomosynthesis provides no additional information for the detection and characterization of breast cysts.

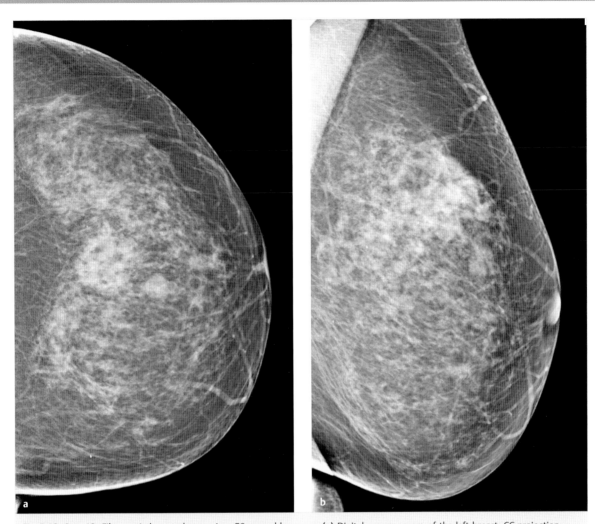

Fig. 5.13 Case 13. Fibrocystic breast changes in a 59-year-old woman. **(a)** Digital mammogram of the left breast, CC projection. **(b)** Digital mammogram of the left breast, MLO projection.

continued ▶

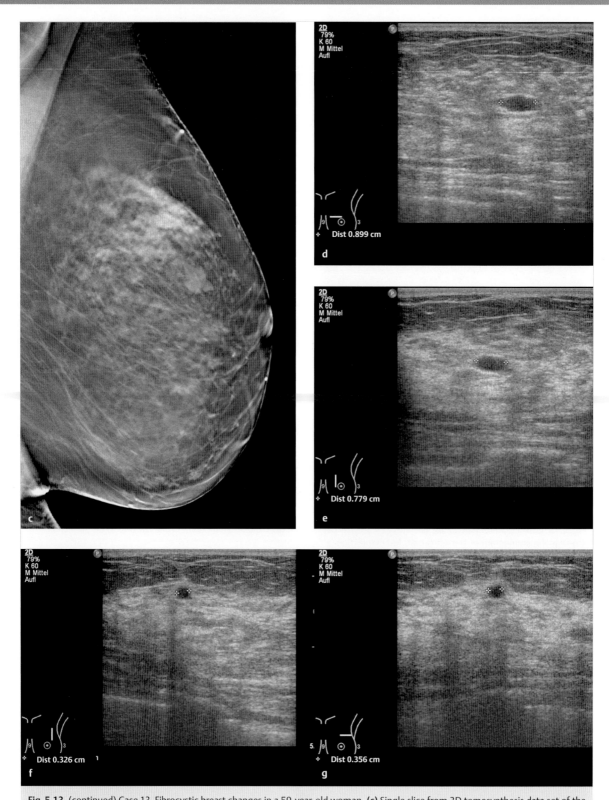

Fig. 5.13 (continued) Case 13. Fibrocystic breast changes in a 59-year-old woman. **(c)** Single slice from 3D tomosynthesis data set of the left breast, MLO projection. **(d)** Ultrasound scan of the mass at the 11 o'clock position (12.5-MHz probe). **(e)** Ultrasound scan of the mass at the 11 o'clock position (12.5-MHz probe), second plane. **(f)** Ultrasound scan of the mass at the 1 o'clock position. **(g)** Ultrasound scan of the left breast mass at the 1 o'clock position, second plane.

5.2.14 Case 14

History

Woman 57 years of age, three children, did not breast-feed. No family history of breast cancer. Left mastodynia has been present for several months. No palpable abnormalities.

Mammography

Right breast: ACR 2. Retroareolar architectural distortion with a subtle spiculated lesion, not visible in the CC view. Scattered microcalcifications. Small, well-circumscribed mass near the chest wall. Classified as BI-RADS 3 (**Fig. 5.14a, c**). Left breast: ACR 2. No masses or suspicious microcalcifications (**Fig. 5.14b, d**).

DBT

MLO view of the right breast shows no evidence of a spiculated lesion or suspicious mass (**Fig. 5.14e**). The small, well-circumscribed mass at skin level is identified as a skin wart (**Fig. 5.14f, Video 5.7**).

Ultrasonography

No evidence of a mass.

Final Diagnosis

Normal findings, classified as BI-RADS 2.

Further Case History

The findings were unchanged at 2-year follow-up.

Discussion

Tomosynthesis can resolve the questionable spiculated lesion on mammography and can accurately localize the well-circumscribed lesion to skin level.

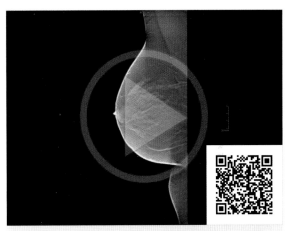

Video 5.7 Case 14. DBT data set of the right breast, MLO projection. Small mass with smooth margins, a wart at skin level.

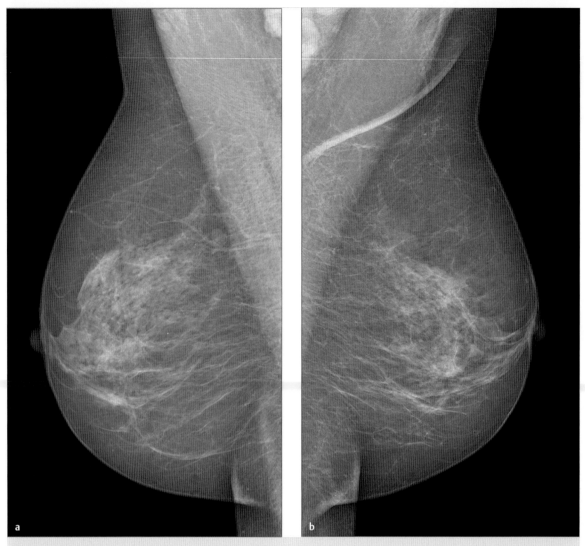

a

b

Fig. 5.14 Case 14. 57-year-old woman with mastodynia. **(a)** Digital mammogram of the right breast, MLO projection. **(b)** Digital mammogram of the left breast, MLO projection.

continued ▶

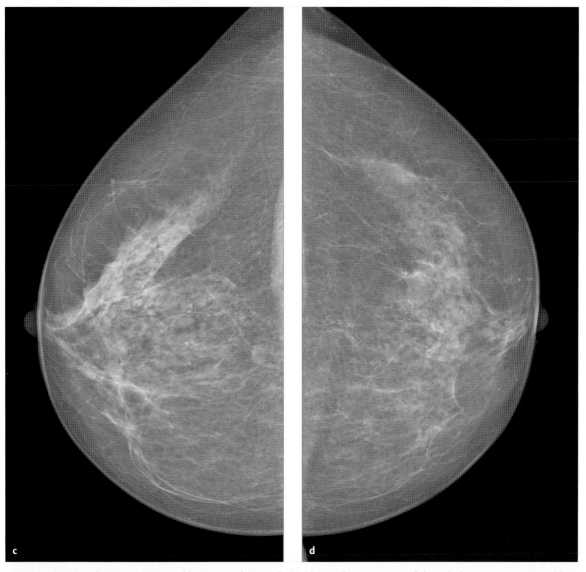

Fig. 5.14 (continued) Case 14. 57-year-old woman with mastodynia. **(c)** Digital mammogram of the right breast, CC projection. **(d)** Digital mammogram of the left breast, CC projection.

continued ▶

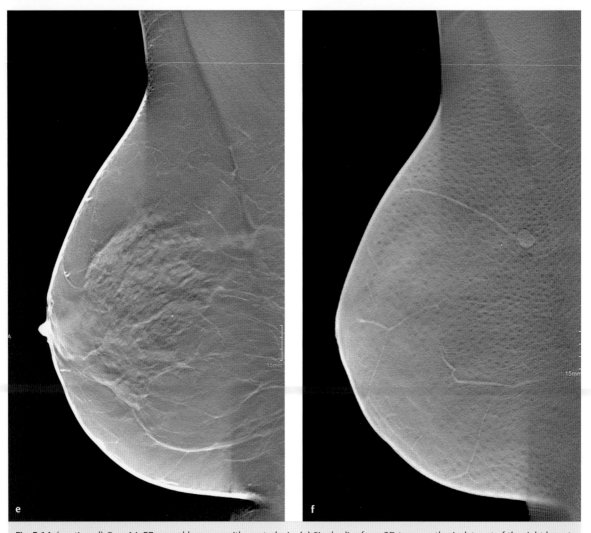

Fig. 5.14 (continued) Case 14. 57-year-old woman with mastodynia. **(e)** Single slice from 3D tomosynthesis data set of the right breast, MLO projection. **(f)** Single slice from 3D tomosynthesis data set of the right breast, MLO projection.

5.2.15 Case 15

History

Woman 48 years of age with no family history of breast cancer, not on hormone therapy. G2, P2, did not breast-feed. Status post-excisional biopsy of the left breast in 1996 with benign histology.

Mammography

Right breast: ACR 3. A benign-appearing lesion is seen in the lower outer quadrant, classified as BI-RADS 2 (**Fig. 5.15a, c**). Left breast: ACR 3. A 1-cm spiculated mass is found in the upper outer quadrant, 5.7 cm from the nipple. It is accompanied by scattered microcalcifications and additional masses whose margins are difficult to evaluate. The spiculated lesion is classified as BI-RADS 4 (**Fig. 5.15b, d**).

DBT

CC view of the left breast shows a 1-cm spiculated mass 6 cm from the nipple, with scattered microcalcifications (**Fig. 5.15e**). Multiple masses with smooth margins are also visible (**Fig. 5.15f, Video 5.8**).

Ultrasonography

Ultrasound scan of the left breast shows an irregularly shaped hypoechoic mass at the 12 o'clock position, measuring 0.9 × 0.5 × 0.7 cm (**Fig. 5.15 g**).

Further Case History

Vacuum biopsy of the mass gave a histologic diagnosis of focal atypical epithelial hyperplasia and an intraductal papilloma. Owing to the B3 classification, the lesions were surgically excised.

Final Diagnosis

Atypical ductal hyperplasia and intraductal papilloma.

Discussion

Tomosynthesis confirms the mammographically suspicious lesion. The other mammographic densities are definitely characterized as benign by DBT.

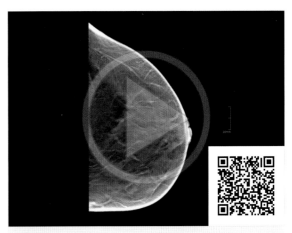

Video 5.8 Case 15. DBT data set of the left breast, CC projection. Multiple smooth-bordered masses plus a 1-cm spiculated mass 6 cm from the nipple, with scattered microcalcifications.

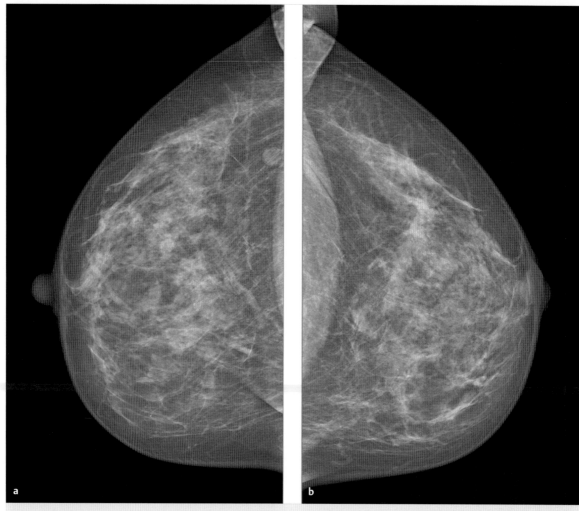

Fig. 5.15 Case 15. 48-year-old woman, status post-excisional biopsy with benign histology. **(a)** Digital mammogram of the right breast, CC projection. **(b)** Digital mammogram of the left breast, CC projection.

continued ▶

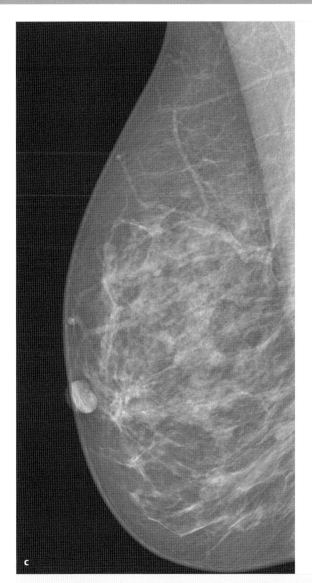
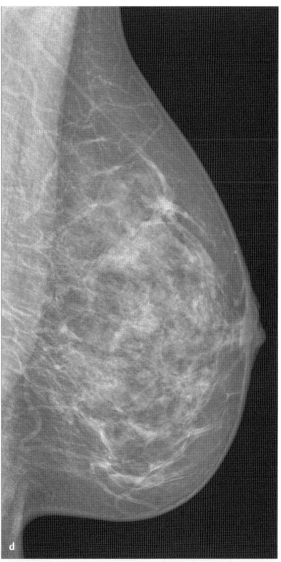

Fig. 5.15 (continued) Case 15. 48-year-old woman, status post-excisional biopsy with benign histology. **(c)** Digital mammogram of the right breast, MLO projection. **(d)** Digital mammogram of the left breast, MLO projection.

continued ▶

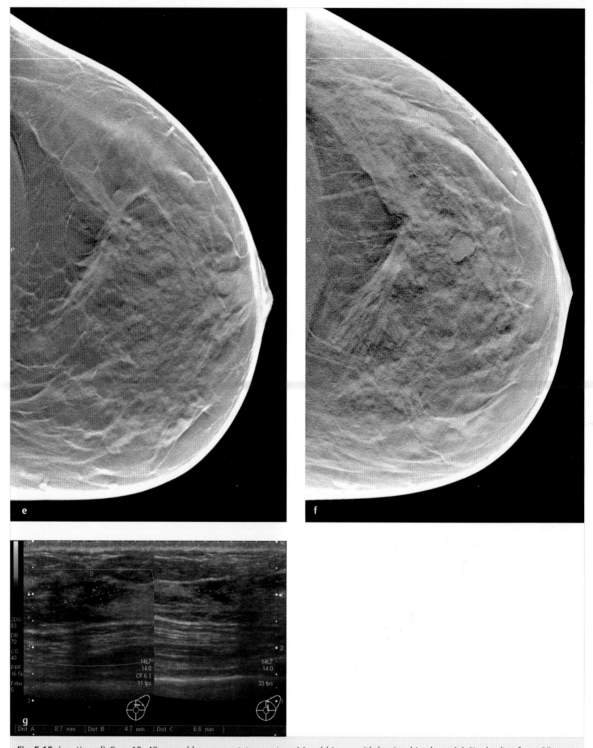

Fig. 5.15 (continued) Case 15. 48-year-old woman, status post-excisional biopsy with benign histology. (e) Single slice from 3D tomosynthesis data set of the left breast, CC projection. (f) Single slice from 3D tomosynthesis data set of the left breast, CC projection. (g) Ultrasound scans of the mass in the left breast.

5.2.16 Case 16

History

Asymptomatic 58-year-old woman with a family history of breast cancer and known significant fibrocystic changes. Both breasts have palpable nodularity but no other abnormalities.

Mammography

Right breast: ACR 4. Nodular pattern of fibrocystic changes with scattered, monomorphic microcalcifications. Suspicious masses are not seen in either the CC or MLO views. Classified as BI-RADS 2 (**Fig. 5.16a, b**).

DBT

MLO view of the right breast shows subtle retroareolar spiculations 2 cm from the nipple, with an associated mass measuring approximately 5 × 5 mm. Classified as BI-RADS 4 (**Fig. 5.16c, d**).

Ultrasonography

Ultrasound scans of the right breast show a periareolar hypoechoic area with ill-defined margins and associated architectural distortion. It measures 5 × 5 × 5 mm. Classified as BI-RADS 5 (**Fig. 5.16e, f**).

Further Case History

Ultrasound-guided core-needle biopsy identified the mass as a grade 1 carcinoma, 5 mm in diameter.

Final Diagnosis

Grade 1 invasive breast carcinoma NST.

Discussion

The spiculated mass is detected by tomosynthesis but not by mammography. The use of 3D tomosynthesis in this case increases sensitivity and allows detection of a breast cancer that is occult on standard mammograms.

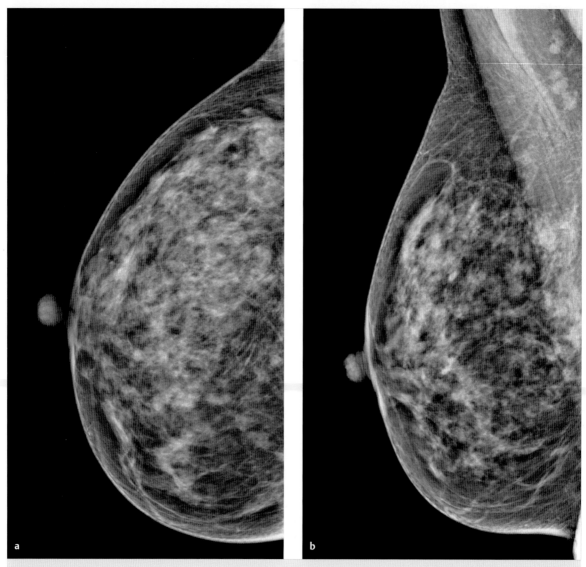

Fig. 5.16 Case 16. 58-year-old woman with significant fibrocystic changes and palpable nodularity in both breasts. **(a)** Digital mammogram of the right breast, CC projection. **(b)** Digital mammogram of the right breast, MLO projection.

continued ▶

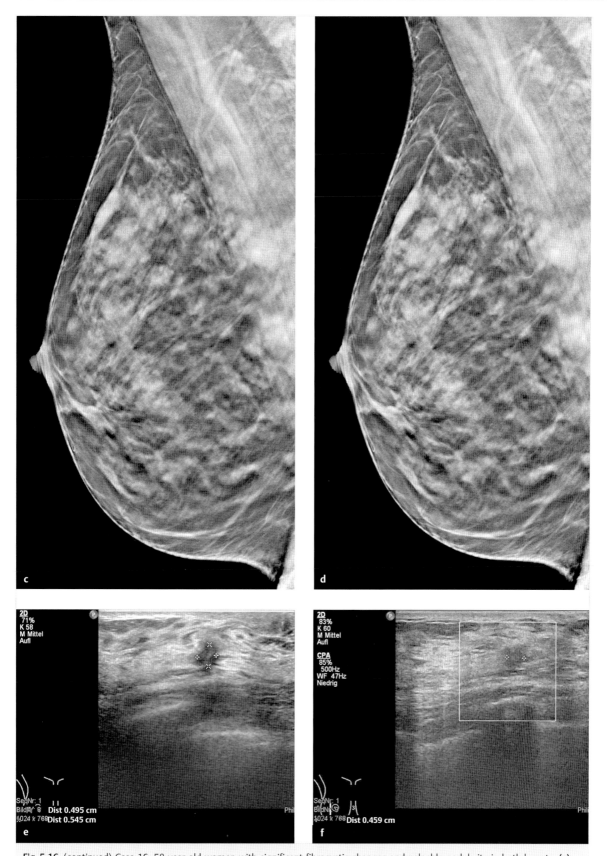

Fig. 5.16 (continued) Case 16. 58-year-old woman with significant fibrocystic changes and palpable nodularity in both breasts. **(c)** Single slice from 3D tomosynthesis data set of the right breast, MLO projection. **(d)** Single slice from 3D tomosynthesis data set of the right breast, MLO projection. **(e)** Ultrasound scan of the mass. **(f)** Ultrasound scan of the mass, second plane.

5.2.17 Case 17

History

Woman 38 years of age with no family history of breast cancer. G2, P2, breastfed both children for 3 months. A progressive, tender mass has been present in the upper outer quadrant of the right breast for several months. A firm, fixed mass measuring 3 × 3 cm is noted in that breast quadrant on physical examination.

Mammography

Right breast: ACR 3. Coarse pattern of fibrocystic changes with scattered, rounded monomorphic microcalcifications. Classified as BI-RADS 2 (**Fig. 5.17a, b**).

DBT

MLO view of the right breast shows marked architectural distortion covering an area of 4 × 3 × 3 cm cranial to the nipple. Classified as BI-RADS 5 (**Fig. 5.17c–e**).

Ultrasonography

Scans of the right breast show a large area of architectural distortion at the 11 to 12 o'clock position that disrupts the Cooper's ligaments and includes ill-defined hypoechoic zones. The area measures 3.7 × 1.5 × 3.6 cm and is suspicious for pectoralis muscle invasion (**Fig. 5.17f, g**).

Further Case History

Ultrasound-guided core-needle biopsy revealed grade 2 invasive lobular carcinoma.

Final Diagnosis

Invasive lobular breast carcinoma.

Discussion

Only tomosynthesis and supplemental ultrasonography show an imaging correlate for the palpable right breast mass. Standard digital mammograms are false negative for this pT 3 lesion. In this case, therefore, tomosynthesis provides greater sensitivity than digital mammography.

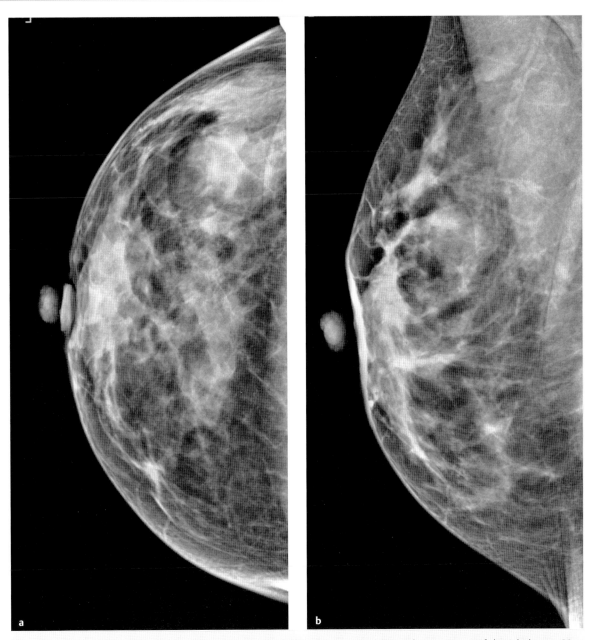

Fig. 5.17 Case 17. 38-year-old woman with a progressive, tender, firm breast mass. **(a)** Digital mammogram of the right breast, CC projection. **(b)** Digital mammogram of the right breast, MLO projection.

continued ▶

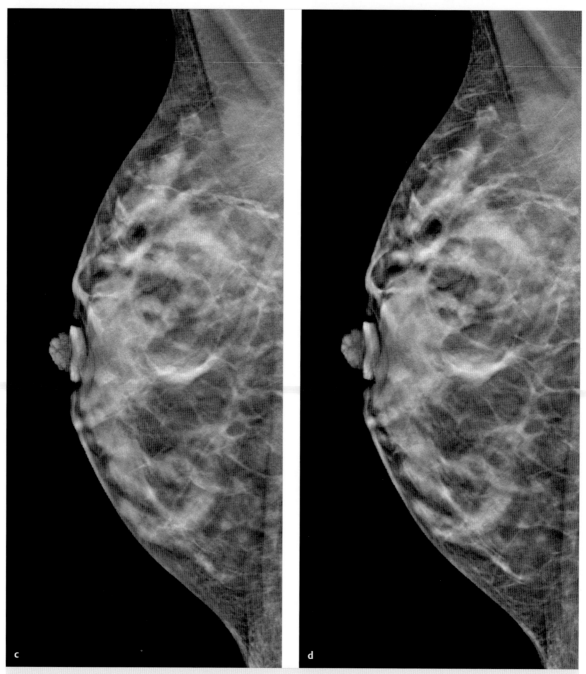

Fig. 5.17 (continued) Case 17. 38-year-old woman with a progressive, tender, firm breast mass. **(c)** Single slice from 3D tomosynthesis data set of the right breast, MLO projection. **(d)** Single slice from 3D tomosynthesis data set of the right breast, MLO projection.

continued ▶

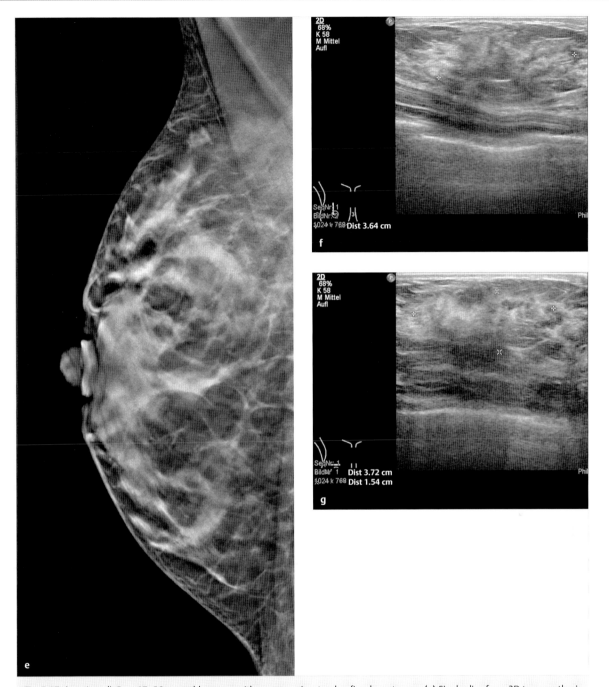

Fig. 5.17 (continued) Case 17. 38-year-old woman with a progressive, tender, firm breast mass. **(e)** Single slice from 3D tomosynthesis data set of the right breast, MLO projection. **(f)** Ultrasound scan of the right breast lesion at the 11 to 12 o'clock position. **(g)** Ultrasound scan of the right breast lesion at the 11 to 12 o'clock position.

5.2.18 Case 18

History

Woman 62 years of age with no family history of breast cancer, not on hormone therapy. Malignant melanoma was removed from the outer half of her right breast in May 2011. In May 2012, the patient felt a nodule in the surgical scar.

Mammography

Right breast: ACR 2. A mass measuring 2.2 × 1.5 × 1.0 cm is visible in the axillary tail. An asymmetric density is also noted in the upper outer quadrant (**Fig. 5.18a, c**). Left breast: ACR 1. Mammograms of the left breast do not show a mass or suspicious microcalcifications (**Fig. 5.18b, d**).

DBT

DBT of the right breast in the CC projection. A mass measuring 2.2 × 1.5 × 1.0 cm is located at the 9 o'clock position in the axillary tail. The asymmetric density in the upper outer quadrant has typical features of heterotopic glandular tissue, with no evidence of malignancy (**Fig. 5.18e, Video 5.9**).

Ultrasonography

Ultrasound scans of the right breast show a richly perfused hypoechoic mass in the axillary tail, infiltrating the surrounding tissue (**Fig. 5.18f**). It measures 2.1 × 1.1 × 1.6 cm and has a slightly hyperechoic rim. No other masses are detected in the right breast.

Further Case History

The palpable mass in the right axillary tail was surgically removed. Based on negative tomosynthesis and normal sonograms, the asymmetric density in the upper outer quadrant of the right breast was not biopsied.

Final Diagnosis

Histology identified the axillary tail lesion as metastatic melanoma. The asymmetric density in the upper outer quadrant remained unchanged over time, confirming the DBT diagnosis.

Discussion

Owing to its high negative predictive value, DBT can increase confidence in the exclusion of breast masses.

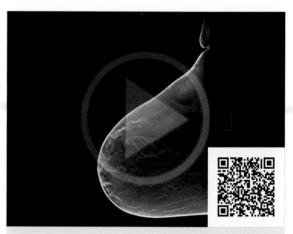

Video 5.9 Case 18. DBT data set of the right breast, CC projection. A mass measuring 2.2 × 1.5 × 1.0 cm is found at the 9 o'clock position in the axillary tail. The asymmetric density in the upper outer quadrant is typical of heterotopic glandular tissue with no evidence of malignancy.

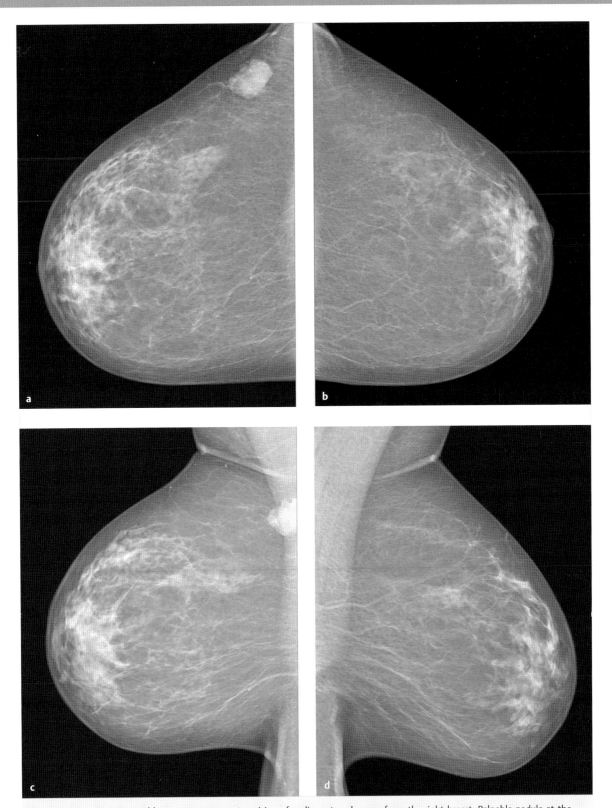

Fig. 5.18 Case 18. 62-year-old woman, status post-excision of malignant melanoma from the right breast. Palpable nodule at the surgical site. **(a)** Digital mammogram of the right breast, CC projection. **(b)** Digital mammogram of the left breast, CC projection. **(c)** Digital mammogram of the right breast, MLO projection. **(d)** Digital mammogram of the left breast, MLO projection.

continued ▶

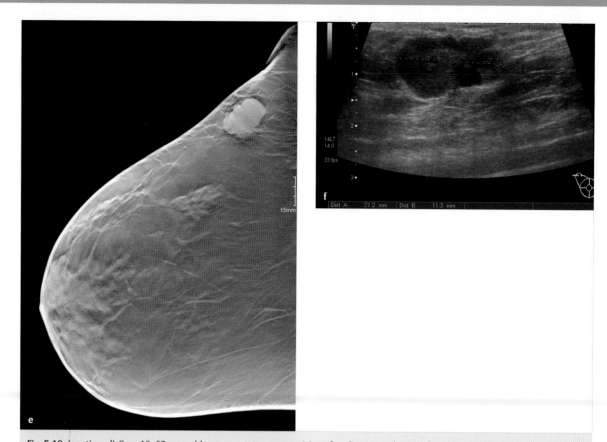

Fig. 5.18 (continued) Case 18. 62-year-old woman, status post-excision of malignant melanoma from the right breast. Palpable nodule at the surgical site. **(e)** Single slice from 3D tomosynthesis data set of the right breast. CC view shows a mass measuring 2.2 × 1.5 × 1.0 cm at the 9 o'clock position in the axillary tail. The asymmetric density in the upper outer quadrant is typical of heterotopic breast parenchyma; no evidence of malignancy. **(f)** Ultrasound scan of the mass in the axillary tail.

5.2.19 Case 19

History

Woman 52 years of age, G2, P2, breastfed both children. She has a family history of breast cancer (maternal aunt and two cousins). She also has a personal history of invasive carcinoma NST in the left breast, first diagnosed in January 2010. She underwent a tumor-adapted left reduction mammoplasty with postoperative radiation, plus a right reduction mammoplasty.

Mammography

Right breast: ACR 2. Mass with ill-defined margins in the upper inner quadrant, measuring 1.2 × 0.8 × 0.9 cm and located 9.6 cm from the nipple. Progressive increased lesion density is noted relative to prior mammograms (**Fig. 5.19e, f**). Multiple axillary lymph nodes. Classified as BI-RADS 4 (**Fig. 5.19a, c**). Left breast: ACR 2. Skin thickening is seen predominantly in the lower breast. Streaky bands of scar tissue are visible in the lower inner quadrant and a calcified oil cyst in the upper breast. Overall classification is BI-RADS 2 (**Fig. 5.19b, d**).

DBT

CC view of the right breast shows a triangular mass with smooth margins in the upper inner quadrant, measuring 0.7 × 0.7 cm and located 10 cm from the nipple (**Fig. 5.19g**). Classified as BI-RADS 2 (**Video 5.10**).

Ultrasonography

Ultrasound scans of the right breast show an apparent correlate of the mass at the 2 o'clock position, measuring 0.5 × 0.8 × 0.6 cm (**Fig. 5.19h**).

Further Case History

The mammographic and sonographic findings warranted recall. Because ultrasonography could not positively reproduce the radiographic findings, stereotactic biopsy was performed.

Final Diagnosis

Tumor-free breast tissue with heavy scarring, old hemorrhages, and small areas of old fat necrosis.

Discussion

The nonsuperimposed tomosynthesis images show that the lesion has sharp margins, creating a lower index of suspicion than mammography. Biopsy was still performed, however, to allow a confident exclusion of malignancy.

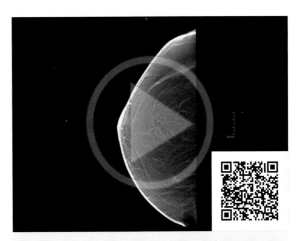

Video 5.10 Case 19. DBT data set of the right breast, CC projection. Triangular mass with smooth margins in the upper inner quadrant. Measures 0.7 × 0.7 cm, located 10 cm from the nipple.

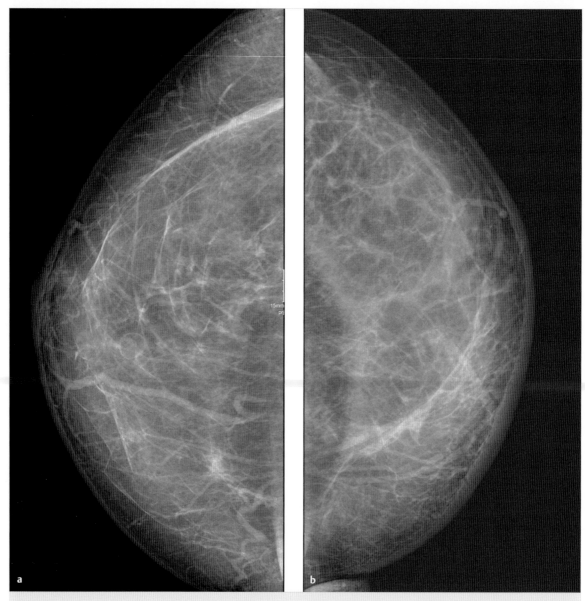

Fig. 5.19 Case 19. 52-year-old woman, status post-invasive carcinoma NST; had a tumor-encompassing left reduction mammoplasty with postoperative radiation and a right reduction mammoplasty. **(a)** Digital mammogram of the right breast, CC projection. **(b)** Digital mammogram of the left breast, CC projection.

continued ▶

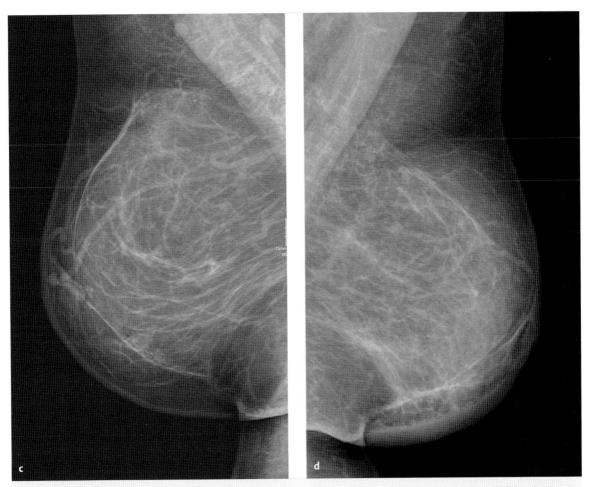

Fig. 5.19 (continued) Case 19. 52-year-old woman, status post-invasive carcinoma NST; had a tumor-encompassing left reduction mammoplasty with postoperative radiation and a right reduction mammoplasty. **(c)** Digital mammogram of the right breast, MLO projection. **(d)** Digital mammogram of the left breast, MLO projection.

continued ▶

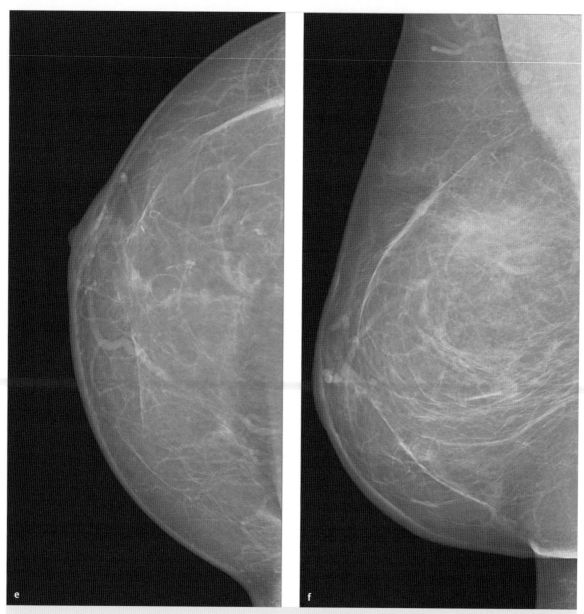

Fig. 5.19 (continued) Case 19. 52-year-old woman, status post-invasive carcinoma NST; had a tumor-encompassing left reduction mammoplasty with postoperative radiation and a right reduction mammoplasty. **(e)** Prior digital mammogram (1 year earlier) of the right breast, CC projection. **(f)** Prior digital mammogram (1 year earlier) of the right breast, MLO projection.

continued ▶

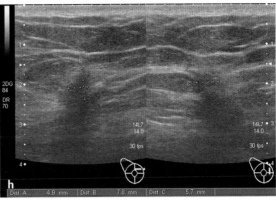

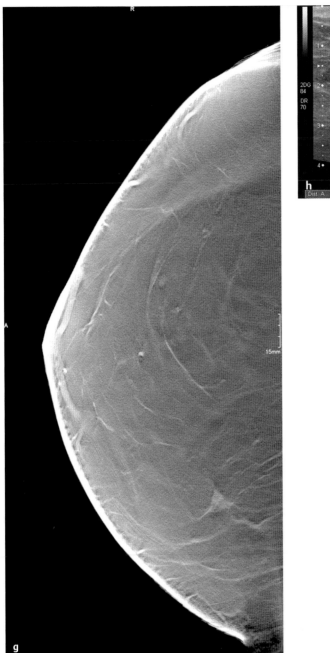

Fig. 5.19 (continued) Case 19. 52-year-old woman, status post-invasive carcinoma NST; had a tumor-encompassing left reduction mammoplasty with postoperative radiation and a right reduction mammoplasty. (g) Single slice from 3D tomosynthesis data set of the right breast, CC projection. (h) Ultrasound scans of the mass.

5.2.20 Case 20

History

Woman 76 years of age, G1, P1, breastfed for 6 months. Well-healed scar from previous left breast-conserving surgery (BCS) for breast cancer in 2009. No palpable masses in either breast. Maternal history of breast cancer at age 80 years. Not currently on hormone therapy.

Mammography

Right breast: ACR 1. Pleomorphic microcalcification cluster at the 12 o'clock position, bordered by a spiculated lesion in the CC projection. No definite correlate in the MLO projection. Classified as BI-RADS 4 (**Fig. 5.20a, c**). Left breast: ACR 1. Known, unchanged microcalcification cluster in the lower central breast. Clip at the 12 o'clock position following BCS for breast cancer in 2009. Classified as BI-RADS 2 (**Fig. 5.20b, d**).

DBT

DBT of the right breast in the CC projection. The microcalcifications are clearly demonstrated by tomosynthesis (**Fig. 5.20e**). The spiculated mammographic lesion at the 12 o'clock position is defined with greater clarity by DBT (**Fig. 5.20f**). Classified as BI-RADS 5 (**Video 5.11**).

Ultrasonography

Architectural distortion is seen at the 12 o'clock position but does not correlate with the spiculated mammographic lesion (**Fig. 5.20g**).

Further Case History

Stereotactic vacuum biopsy of the spiculated lesion at the 12 o'clock position in the right breast revealed solid papillary carcinoma.

Final Diagnosis

Solid papillary carcinoma.

Discussion

The spiculated mass is defined more clearly by tomosynthesis than conventional mammography and can be positively distinguished from a summation artifact.

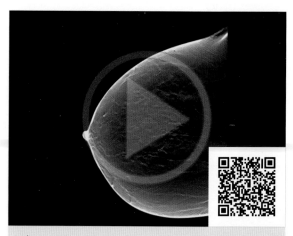

Video 5.11 Case 20. DBT data set of the right breast, CC projection. Spiculated mass and microcalcifications.

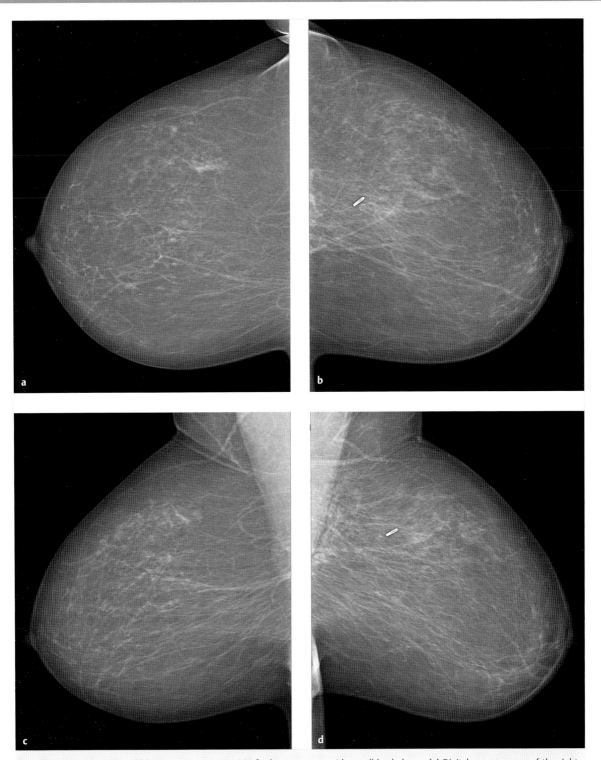

Fig. 5.20 Case 20. 76-year-old woman, status post-BCS for breast cancer with a well-healed scar. **(a)** Digital mammogram of the right breast, CC projection. **(b)** Digital mammogram of the left breast, CC projection. **(c)** Digital mammogram of the right breast, MLO projection. **(d)** Digital mammogram of the left breast, MLO projection.

continued ▶

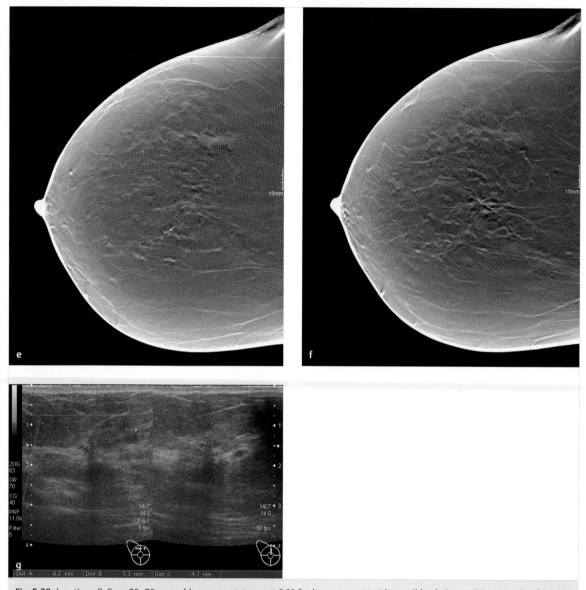

Fig. 5.20 (continued) Case 20. 76-year-old woman, status post-BCS for breast cancer with a well-healed scar. **(e)** Single slice from 3D tomosynthesis data set of the right breast, CC projection. Microcalcifications. **(f)** Single slice from 3D tomosynthesis data set of the right breast, CC projection. Spiculated lesion. **(g)** Ultrasound scans of the suspicious area.

5.2.21 Case 21

History

Asymptomatic 65-year-old woman, seen 5 years after BCS for breast cancer (tumor stage pT 1 c N0 M0). Clinical examination shows a well-healed scar and tissue defect at the 2 o'clock position in the left breast, with otherwise normal findings.

Mammography

Left breast: ACR 3. Architectural distortion at the 2 o'clock position after BCS, 6 cm from the nipple. Also small areas of lipoid necrosis. The finding is interpreted as a postoperative scar. Classified as BI-RADS 2 (**Fig. 5.21a, b**).

DBT

DBT of the left breast in the MLO projection. Tomosynthesis clearly displays the excision scar as an architectural distortion at the 2 o'clock position. The small areas of lipoid necrosis at the surgery site are also well defined. No suspicious masses are seen (**Fig. 5.21c, d**).

Final Diagnosis

Scar after BCS, BI-RADS 2.

Discussion

3D tomosynthesis clearly depicts the scar and architectural distortion following BCS. Despite the dense parenchymal structures, the volume data set can positively exclude a mass in or adjacent to the surgical scar.

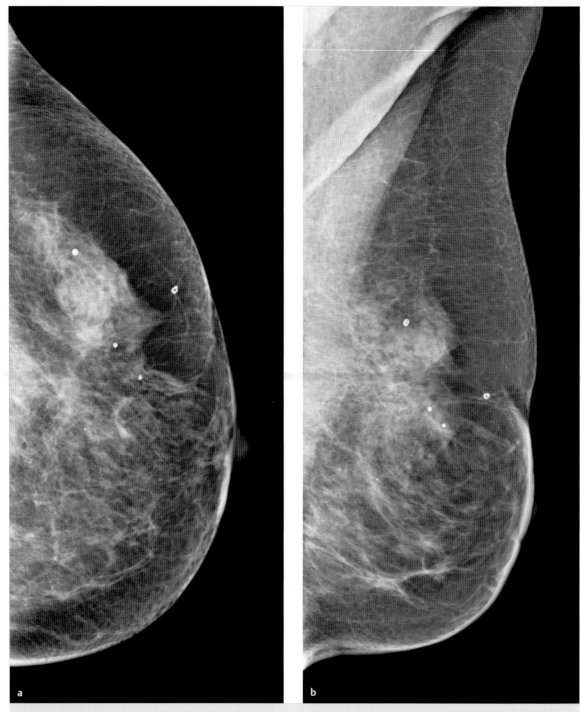

Fig. 5.21 Case 21. 65-year-old woman, status post-BCS for breast cancer with a well-healed scar and tissue defect. (a) Digital mammogram of the left breast, CC projection. (b) Digital mammogram of the left breast, MLO projection.

continued ▶

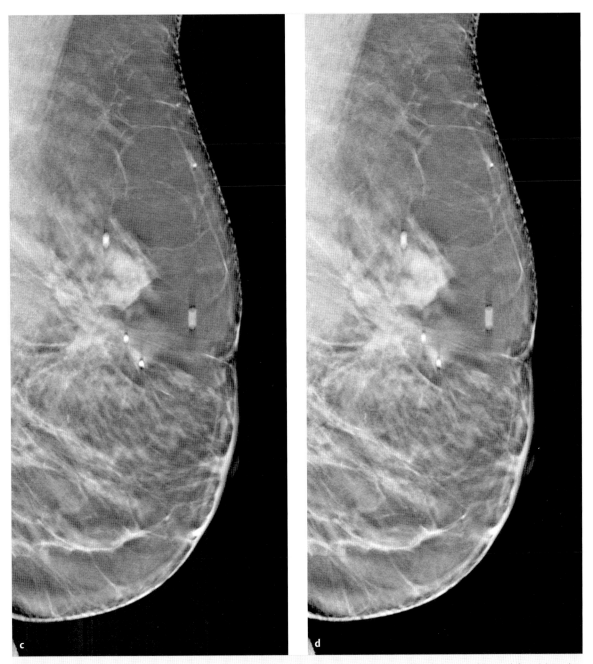

Fig. 5.21 (continued) Case 21. 65-year-old woman, status post-BCS for breast cancer with a well-healed scar and tissue defect. **(c)** Single slice from 3D tomosynthesis data set of the left breast, MLO projection. **(d)** Single slice from 3D tomosynthesis data set of the left breast, MLO projection.

5.2.22 Case 22

History

Asymptomatic 74-year-old woman 8 years after local excision of breast cancer (tumor stage pT 1 a N0 M0). Normal physical findings except for a well-healed scar and known tissue defect at the 4 o'clock position in the right breast.

Mammography

Right breast: ACR 3. CC projection shows a scar with architectural distortion in the inner half of the breast, 4 cm from the nipple. An adjacent questionable density is difficult to evaluate in a projection slightly different from prior mammograms 1 year earlier (**Fig. 5.22b, c**). Classified as BI-RADS 4 (**Fig. 5.22a**). A supplemental CC spot compression view does not completely resolve the suspicious area (**Fig. 5.22d**).

DBT

CC and MLO views of the right breast demonstrate a spiculated mass measuring 7 × 6 mm, in the scarred area. The lesion is highly suspicious for a scar recurrence and is classified as BI-RADS 5 (**Fig. 5.22e, f**).

Ultrasonography

The scar is bordered by a hyperechoic mass, 7 × 5 × 4 mm, with ill-defined margins. Classified as BI-RADS 5 (**Fig. 5.22g, h**).

Further Case History

Ultrasound-guided core-needle biopsy identified the mass as a 6-mm grade 2 carcinoma, interpreted histologically as a scar recurrence.

Final Diagnosis

Scar recurrence, postoperative tumor stage T1 b.

Discussion

The standard mammograms and spot compression view show only a subtle area of increased density in the scarred area. Tomosynthesis images in both the CC and MLO projections reveal a spiculated mass. DBT in this case adds information to the mammograms and spot view and permits definite detection of the scar recurrence.

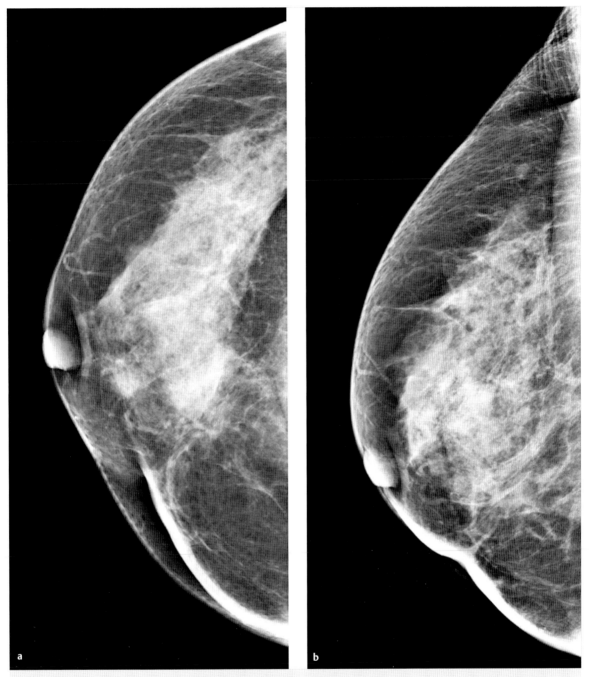

Fig. 5.22 Case 22. 74-year-old woman, status post-BCS for breast cancer with a well-healed scar and tissue defect. **(a)** Digital mammogram of the right breast, CC projection. **(b)** Prior digital mammogram (1 year earlier) of the right breast, CC projection.

continued ▶

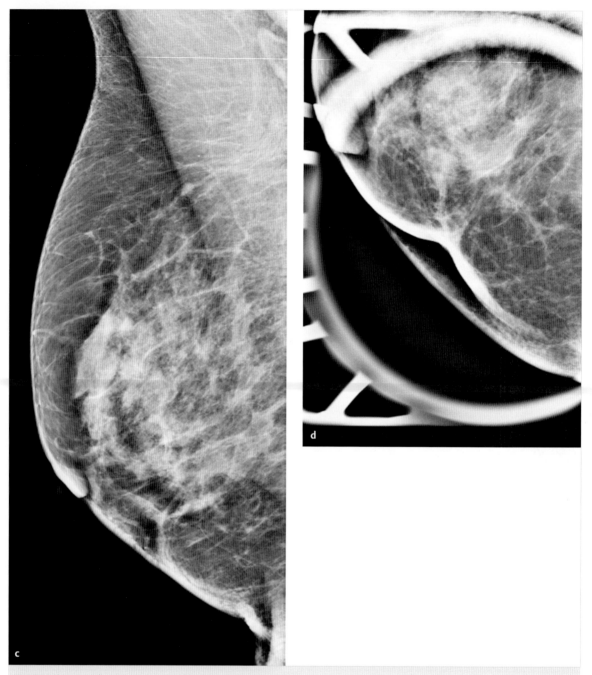

Fig. 5.22 (continued) Case 22. 74-year-old woman, status post-BCS for breast cancer with a well-healed scar and tissue defect. **(c)** Prior digital mammogram (1 year earlier) of the right breast, MLO projection. **(d)** Spot compression view of the right breast, CC projection.
continued ▶

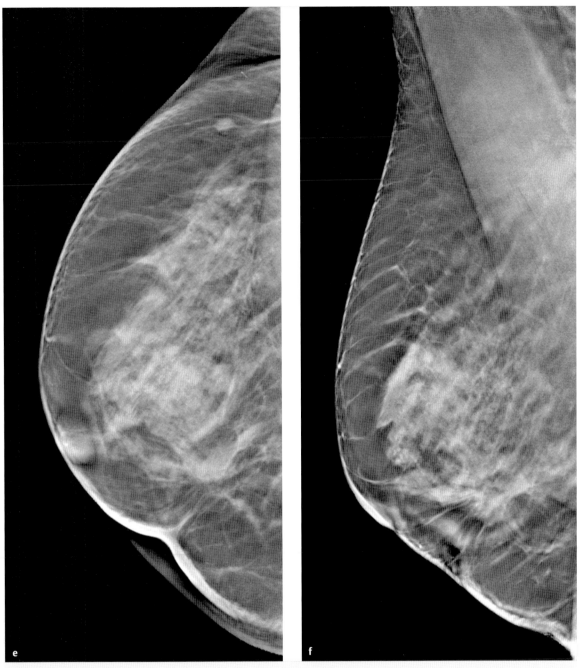

Fig. 5.22 (continued) Case 22. 74-year-old woman, status post-BCS for breast cancer with a well-healed scar and tissue defect. **(e)** Single slice from 3D tomosynthesis data set of the right breast, CC projection. **(f)** Single slice from 3D tomosynthesis data set of the right breast, MLO projection.

continued ▶

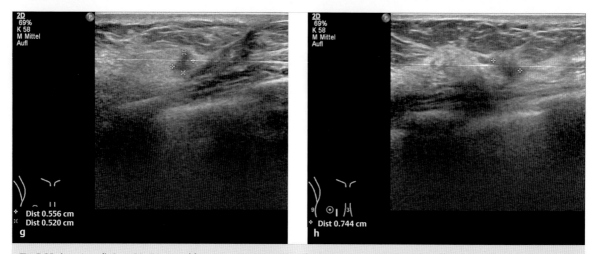

Fig. 5.22 (continued) Case 22. 74-year-old woman, status post-BCS for breast cancer with a well-healed scar and tissue defect. **(g)** Ultrasound scan of the mass. **(h)** Ultrasound scan of the mass, second plane.

5.2.23 Case 23

History

Woman 71 years of age, 3 years after undergoing left BCS for pT 1 b N0 M0 breast cancer. She is asymptomatic with a well-healed scar and tissue defect at the 2 o'clock position in the left breast. She has a tender, movable 1-cm axillary mass, known to have been present since her operation.

Mammography

Left breast: ACR 2. CC view shows a scar with architectural distortion in the outer half of the breast, 7 cm from the nipple. No evidence of a mass. Classified as BI-RADS 2 (**Fig. 5.23a**).

DBT

DBT of the left breast in the MLO projection. Two 4-mm lucent lesions with smooth margins, interpreted as oil cysts, are visible at the 2 o'clock position in the scarred area. Two similar lesions, measuring 7 mm and 13 mm, are visible in the axillary tail and are also interpreted as oil cysts. DBT additionally shows a rounded, prepectoral mass of 7 × 7 mm, with smooth margins. This finding, unchanged for more than 2 years, is interpreted as a reactive lymph node. Classified as BI-RADS 2 (**Fig. 5.23b**).

Ultrasonography

On ultrasonography, the oil cyst in the scarred area appears as a 5-mm mass with smooth margins and mixed echogenicity (**Fig. 5.23c**). Ultrasonography can also detect the oil cysts in the axillary tail (**Fig. 5.23d**). The mass that, on mammography, is presumed to be a lymph node measures 7 × 5 mm by ultrasonography, and has a thickened hypoechoic cortex and a small hilar echo. Its sonographic appearance has been unchanged for more than 2 years (**Fig. 5.23e**).

Final Diagnosis

BI-RADS 2, postoperative scar, oil cysts, and a reactive lymph node.

Discussion

Follow-up in this case relied on a combination of mammography in the CC projection and DBT in the MLO projection. Tomosynthesis permits the accurate characterization of all lesions in the scarred area, all of which are classified as benign (BI-RADS 2).

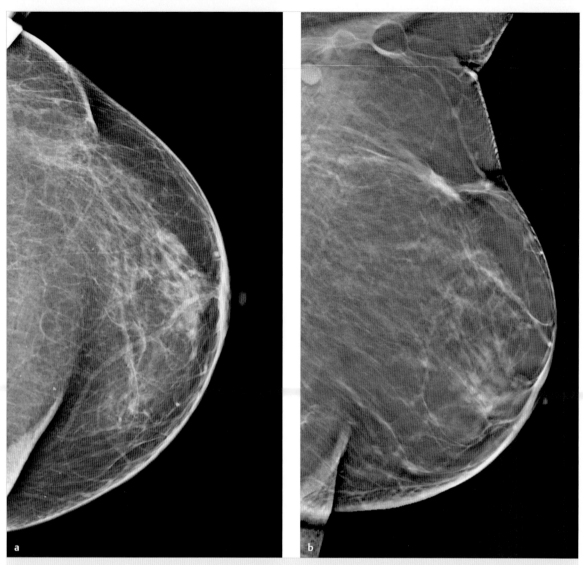

Fig. 5.23 Case 23. 71-year-old woman, status post-BCS for breast cancer with a well-healed scar and tissue defect. Tender, movable axillary mass present since surgery. **(a)** Digital mammogram of the left breast, CC projection. **(b)** Single slice from 3D tomosynthesis data set of the left breast, MLO projection.

continued ▶

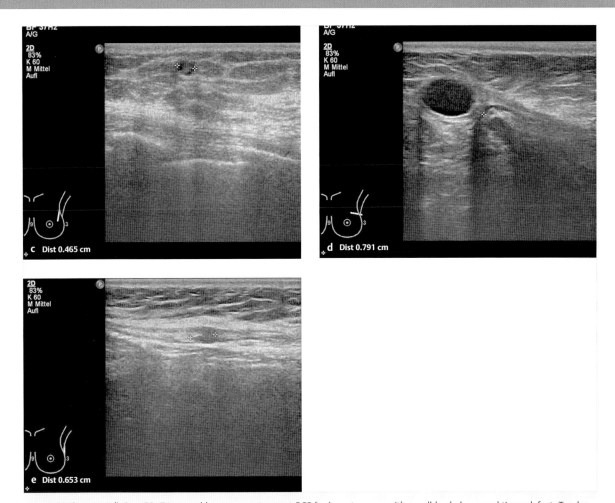

Fig. 5.23 (continued) Case 23. 71-year-old woman, status post-BCS for breast cancer with a well-healed scar and tissue defect. Tender, movable axillary mass present since surgery. **(c)** Ultrasound scan of an oil cyst in the scarred area. **(d)** Ultrasound scan of an oil cyst in the axilla. **(e)** Ultrasound scan of the prepectoral lymph node.

5.2.24 Case 24

History

Woman 59 years of age, G2, P2, breastfed both children for 6 months. Status 5 years post-BCS of the left breast for invasive carcinoma NST, grade 3, pT 1 b (6 mm) pN0 M0. Adjuvant endocrine treatment with anastrozole. Core-needle biopsy of indeterminate sonographic lesion in the left breast 3 years earlier showed sclerosing adenosis with associated microcalcifications.

Mammography

Left breast: ACR 3. At the 12 to 1 o'clock position, 6 cm from the nipple, is an area of scarring and architectural distortion with dystrophic calcifications and typical lipo-necrosis measuring $1.6 \times 1.4 \times 1.6$ cm (**Fig. 5.24a**). Caudal to the liponecrosis is an oblong density measuring 10×3 mm in the MLO projection, classified as BI-RADS 4 (**Fig. 5.24b**). Additional ML mammogram looks normal in that area, suggesting that the suspicious lesion is a summation artifact (**Fig. 5.24c**).

DBT

MLO view of the left breast demonstrates a scar with architectural distortion and a typical oil cyst located 6 cm from the nipple. Dystrophic calcifications are also visible. Tomosynthesis positively identifies the suspicious mammographic density as a summation artifact caused by superimposed parenchyma. Classified as BI-RADS 2 (**Fig. 5.24d–f**).

Ultrasonography

Ultrasound scan of the left breast shows architectural distortion from the skin to chest wall, due to scarring (**Fig. 5.24g**). The scarred area contains typical oil cysts, the largest measuring $15 \times 11 \times 10$ mm (**Fig. 5.24h**).

Final Diagnosis

Summation artifact, BI-RADS 2.

Discussion

The suspicious density in the mammographic oblique view is positively identified by tomosynthesis as a summation artifact. In this case, the combination of mammography in the CC projection and tomosynthesis in the MLO projection would have been sufficient to confirm the diagnosis. To date, no clinical studies have been done on the diagnostic accuracy of complementary-view mammography and DBT after BCS.

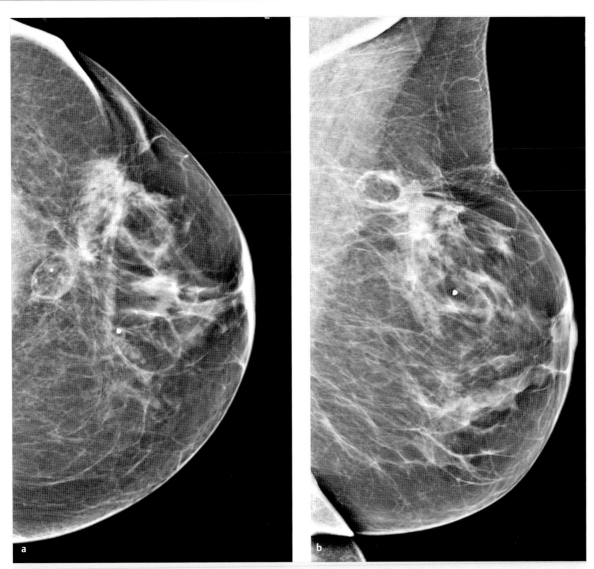

Fig. 5.24 Case 24. 59-year-old woman, status post-BCS for invasive carcinoma NST. Core-needle biopsy shows sclerosing adenosis with associated microcalcifications. **(a)** Digital mammogram of the left breast, CC projection. **(b)** Digital mammogram of the left breast, MLO projection.

continued ▶

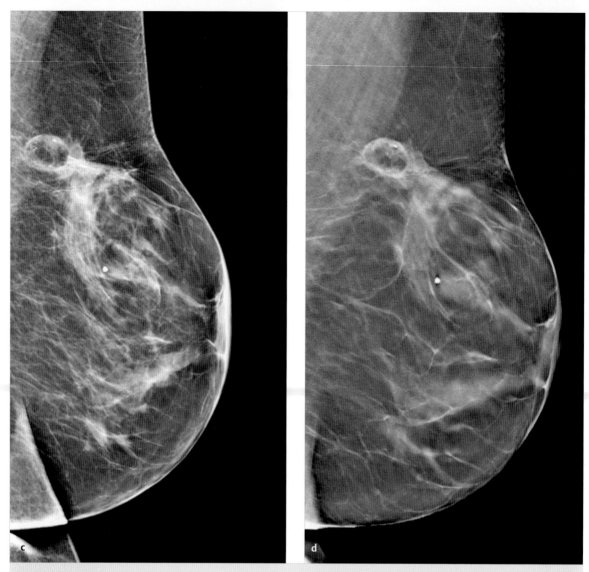

Fig. 5.24 (continued) Case 24. 59-year-old woman, status post-BCS for invasive carcinoma NST. Core-needle biopsy shows sclerosing adenosis with associated microcalcifications. **(c)** Digital mammogram of the left breast in the ML projection. **(d)** Single slice from 3D tomosynthesis data set of the left breast, MLO projection.

continued ▶

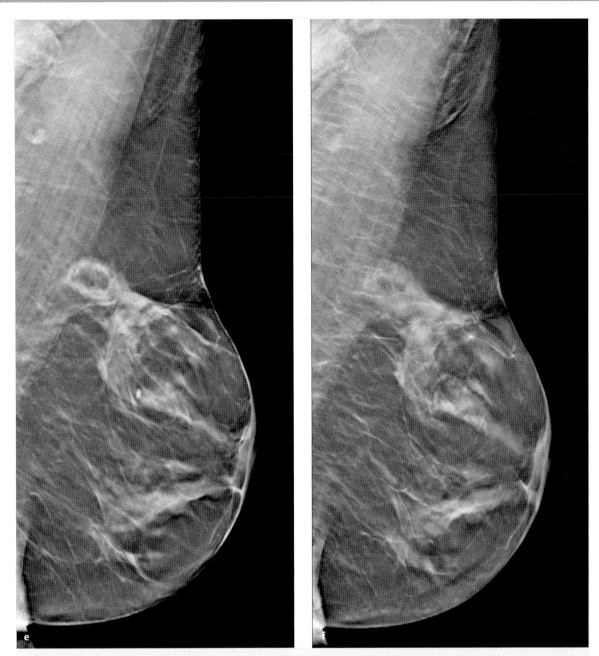

Fig. 5.24 (continued) Case 24. 59-year-old woman, status post-BCS for invasive carcinoma NST. Core-needle biopsy shows sclerosing adenosis with associated microcalcifications. **(e)** Single slice from 3D tomosynthesis data set of the left breast, MLO projection. **(f)** Single slice from 3D tomosynthesis data set of the left breast, MLO projection.

continued ▶

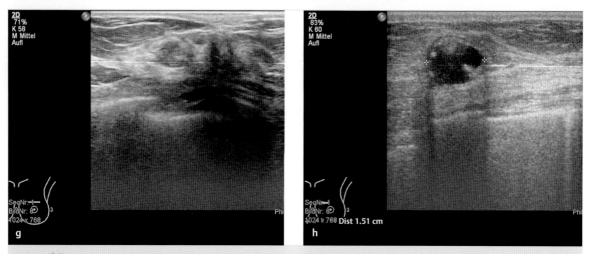

Fig. 5.24 (continued) Case 24. 59-year-old woman, status post-BCS for invasive carcinoma NST. Core-needle biopsy shows sclerosing adenosis with associated microcalcifications. **(g)** Ultrasound scan of the scar. **(h)** Ultrasound scan of an oil cyst.

5.2.25 Case 25

History

Woman 32 years of age, with a palpable mass in the upper outer quadrant of the right breast. G1, P1, breastfed for 10 months. She had a grandmother with breast cancer at age 73 years and an aunt diagnosed with breast cancer at age 45 years. The patient is on hormonal contraception.

Mammography

Right breast: ACR 2. Asymmetry and architectural distortion in the upper outer quadrant. Overall size approximately 3 cm, located 10 cm from the nipple. Classified as BI-RADS 5 (**Fig. 5.25a, c**). Left breast: ACR 2. No mammographic lesion. Lipoid necrosis, classified as BI-RADS 2 (**Fig. 5.25b, d**).

DBT

CC view of the right breast shows a spiculated density measuring 3.2 × 2.8 cm, located 11 cm from the nipple (**Fig. 5.25e**). Adjacent to (**Fig. 5.25f**) and within the density (**Fig. 5.25g**) are multiple well-circumscribed masses, presumably cysts (**Video 5.12**).

Ultrasonography

Scan through the upper outer quadrant of the right breast shows an irregular area with multiple hypoechoic, smooth-bordered lesions that are interpreted as cysts. The area measures 3.4 × 3.0 cm (**Fig. 5.25h**).

Further Case History

Initial ultrasound-guided core-needle biopsy showed only fibrocystic changes. Based on the suspicious mammographic finding, however, it was decided to proceed with local excision.

Final Diagnosis

Ordinary ductal hyperplasia, fibrocystic changes, apocrine metaplasia and adenosis. No evidence of malignancy.

Discussion

Fibrocystic changes may appear as spiculated lesions on mammography and tomosynthesis. In the present case, tomosynthesis confirms the mammographic finding and defines the multiple cysts more clearly than mammograms. On the other hand, DBT in this case does not add information that would have changed the diagnostic work-up.

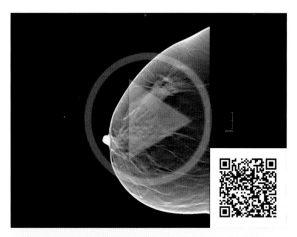

Video 5.12 Case 25. DBT data set of the right breast, CC projection. Spiculated density, 3.2 × 2.8 cm, located 11 cm from the nipple. Within and adjacent to the density are multiple well-circumscribed masses, presumably cysts.

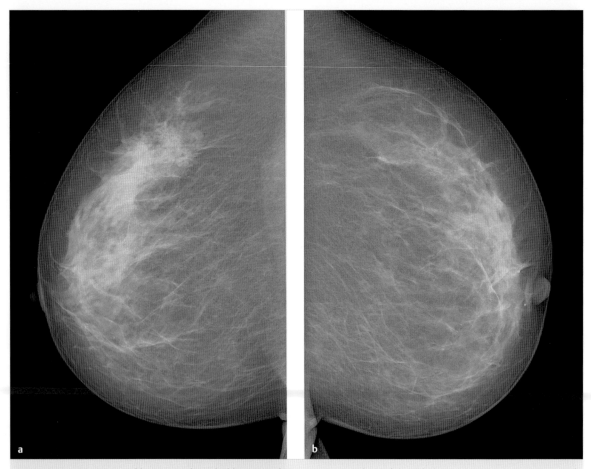

Fig. 5.25 Case 25. 32-year-old woman with a palpable mass in the upper outer quadrant of the right breast. **(a)** Digital mammogram of the right breast, CC projection. **(b)** Digital mammogram of the left breast, CC projection.

continued ▶

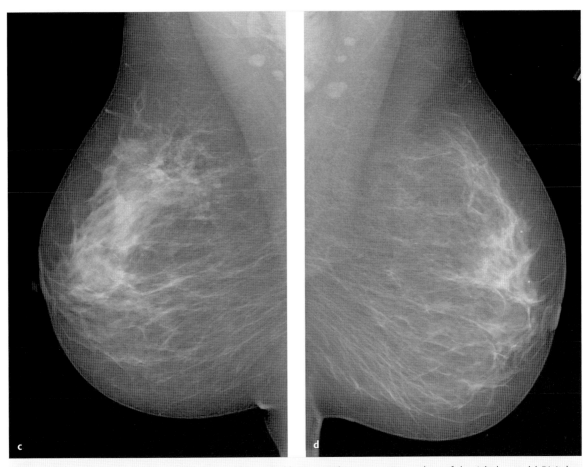

Fig. 5.25 (continued) Case 25. 32-year-old woman with a palpable mass in the upper outer quadrant of the right breast. **(c)** Digital mammogram of the right breast, MLO projection. **(d)** Digital mammogram of the left breast, MLO projection.

continued ▶

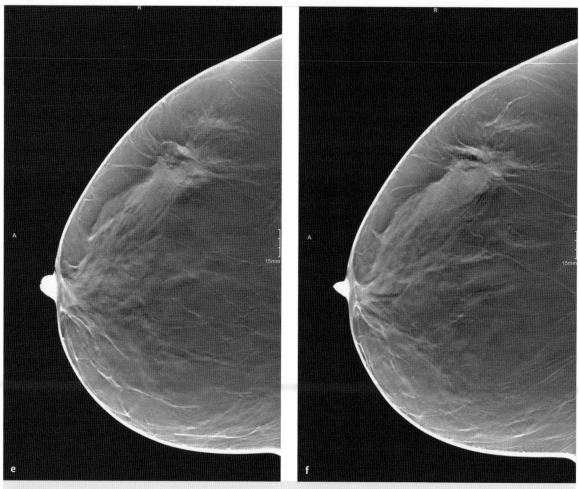

Fig. 5.25 (continued) Case 25. 32-year-old woman with a palpable mass in the upper outer quadrant of the right breast. (e) Single slice from 3D tomosynthesis data set of the right breast, CC projection. (f) Single slice from 3D tomosynthesis data set of the right breast, CC projection.

continued ▶

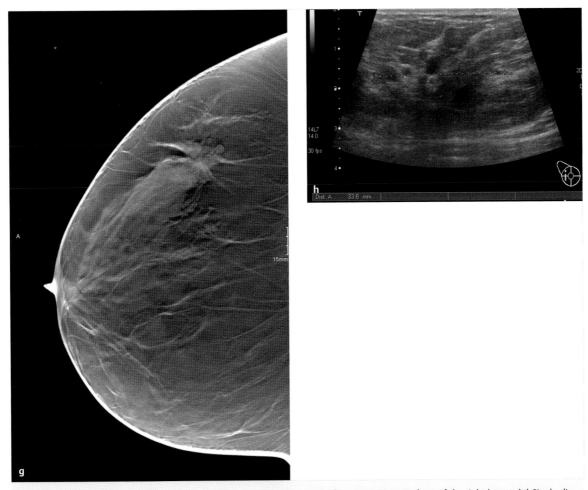

Fig. 5.25 (continued) Case 25. 32-year-old woman with a palpable mass in the upper outer quadrant of the right breast. **(g)** Single slice from 3D tomosynthesis data set of the right breast, CC projection. **(h)** Ultrasound scan of the mass.

5.2.26 Case 26

History

Woman 50 years of age. G2, P2, breastfed for 3 months and 1 year. Not on hormone therapy. Has a sister diagnosed with breast cancer at age 41 years. Patient had a breast cyst resection in 1984, later noticed areas of firmness at the surgical site.

Mammography

Right breast: ACR 2. Density in the upper outer quadrant, 7 cm from the nipple. Classified as BI-RADS 4 (**Fig. 5.26a, c**). Left breast: ACR 2. No masses or microcalcifications. Classified as BI-RADS 2 (**Fig. 5.26b, d**).

DBT

MLO view of the right breast demonstrates a mass measuring 1.9 × 1.5 cm in the upper outer quadrant, located 7 cm from the nipple. The lesion has radiating spicules and a dense center (**Fig. 5.26e**). Classified as BI-RADS 4 (**Video 5.13**).

Ultrasonography

No evidence of a mass.

Further Case History

Stereotactic biopsy yielded tumor-free breast tissue with fibrocystic changes, ordinary ductal hyperplasia, and sclerosing adenosis, classified as a B2 lesion. Based on the suspicious mammographic and tomosynthesis findings, stereotactic wire localization was performed under tomosynthesis guidance, followed by surgical excision for definitive evaluation of the spiculated mass.

Final Diagnosis

Lobular intraepithelial neoplasia (LIN) 2 lesion and fibrocystic changes with focal sclerosing adenosis.

Discussion

This case illustrates the high sensitivity of tomosynthesis in the detection of spiculated lesions. This enables DBT to detect premalignant lesions, although false-positive findings are a possibility. DBT does permit a detailed evaluation of spiculated lesions, however, and future studies may define new morphologic criteria for differentiating malignant and benign lesions by tomosynthesis.

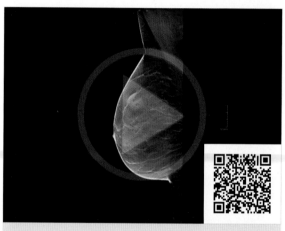

Video 5.13 Case 26. DBT data set of the right breast, MLO projection. A mass measuring 1.9 × 1.5 cm is detected in the upper outer quadrant of the right breast, 7 cm from the nipple. The lesion has radiating spicules and a dense center.

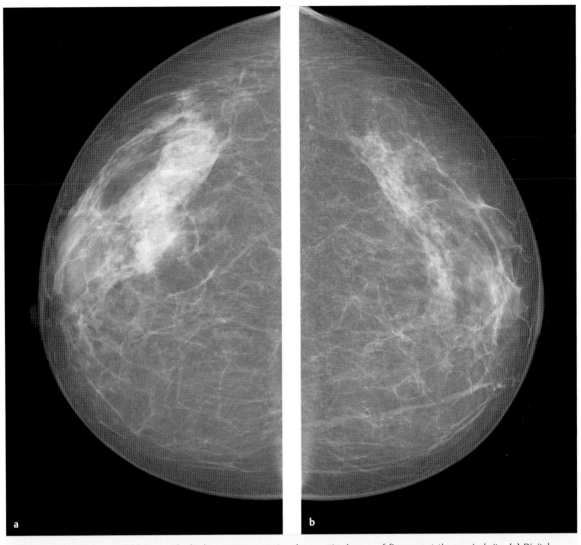

Fig. 5.26 Case 26. 50-year-old woman had a breast cyst resection, later noticed areas of firmness at the surgical site. **(a)** Digital mammogram of the right breast, CC projection. **(b)** Digital mammogram of the left breast, CC projection.

continued ▶

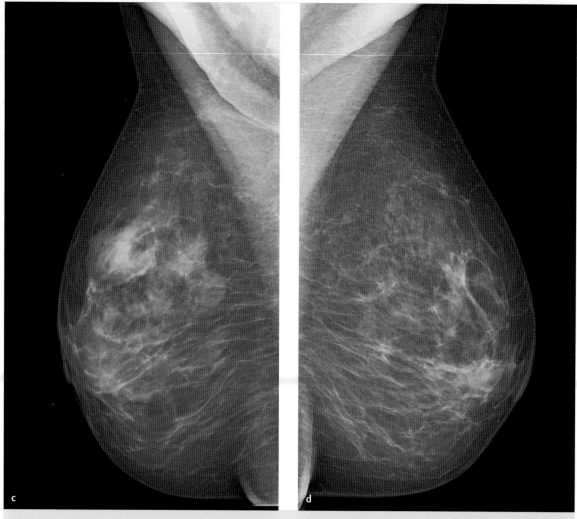

Fig. 5.26 (continued) Case 26. 50-year-old woman had a breast cyst resection, later noticed areas of firmness at the surgical site. **(c)** Digital mammogram of the right breast, MLO projection. **(d)** Digital mammogram of the left breast, MLO projection.

continued ▶

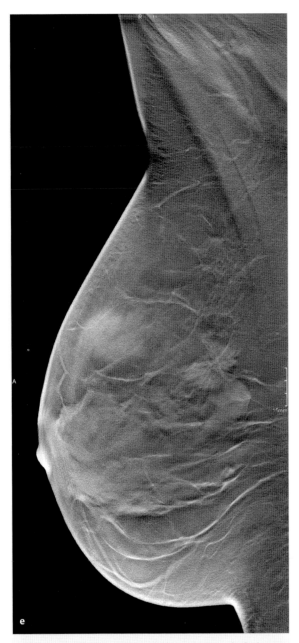

Fig. 5.26 (continued) Case 26. 50-year-old woman had a breast cyst resection, later noticed areas of firmness at the surgical site. **(e)** Single slice from 3D tomosynthesis data set of the right breast, MLO projection. Spiculated lesion.

5.2.27 Case 27

History

Woman 48 years of age, nulliparous. No family history of breast cancer. Patient was on hormonal contraception until 6 years earlier.

Mammography

Right breast: ACR 4. No masses or suspicious microcalcifications. Classified as BI-RADS 2 (**Fig.5.27a, c**). Left breast: ACR 4. Prepectoral microcalcification cluster in the medial half of the breast. Classified as BI-RADS 4 (**Fig. 5.27b, d**).

DBT

CC view of the left breast shows a prepectoral area of architectural distortion, 1.5 cm in size, along with multiple clusters of amorphous microcalcifications. Distance from the nipple is 9 cm (**Fig. 5.27e, f, Video 5.14**).

Ultrasonography

No evidence of a mass.

Further Case History

Stereotactically guided vacuum biopsy of the suspicious area yielded glandular breast tissue with fibrocystic changes, microcalcifications, and columnar cell metaplasia.

Final Diagnosis

Fibrocystic changes with no evidence of malignancy.

Discussion

Microcalcifications are clearly visualized by both mammography and tomosynthesis. DBT slices can map the spatial distribution of the microcalcifications. Clustered microcalcifications are not always found within one slice, however, and this can make it difficult to perceive the calcifications as a cluster. Tomosynthesis does not add information on microcalcification morphology beyond that supplied by mammograms.

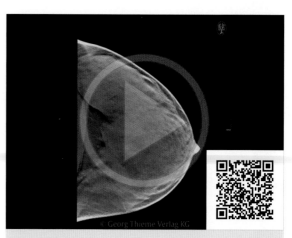

Video 5.14 Case 27. DBT data set of the left breast, CC projection. Prepectoral 1.5-cm area of architectural distortion and multiple clusters of amorphous microcalcifications. Distance from nipple is 9 cm.

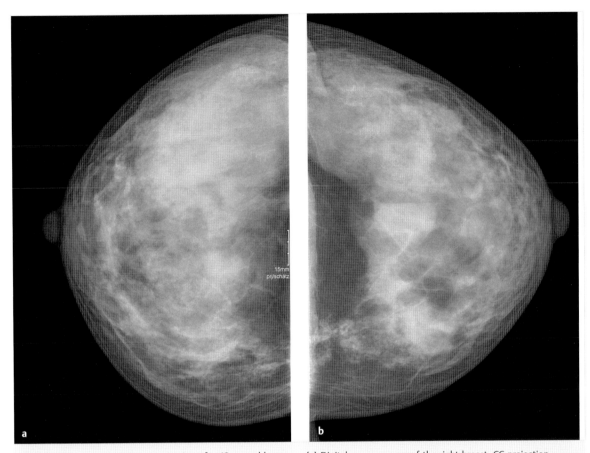

Fig. 5.27 Case 27. Screening examination of a 48-year-old woman. **(a)** Digital mammogram of the right breast, CC projection. **(b)** Digital mammogram of the left breast, CC projection.

continued ▶

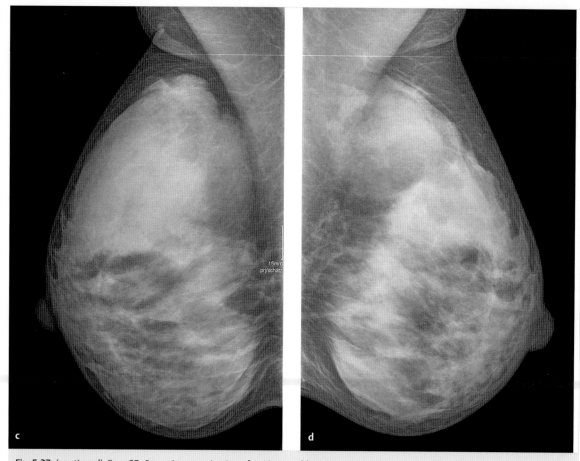

15mm
prj/schätz

c

d

Fig. 5.27 (continued) Case 27. Screening examination of a 48-year-old woman. **(c)** Digital mammogram of the right breast, MLO projection. **(d)** Digital mammogram of the left breast, MLO projection.

continued ▶

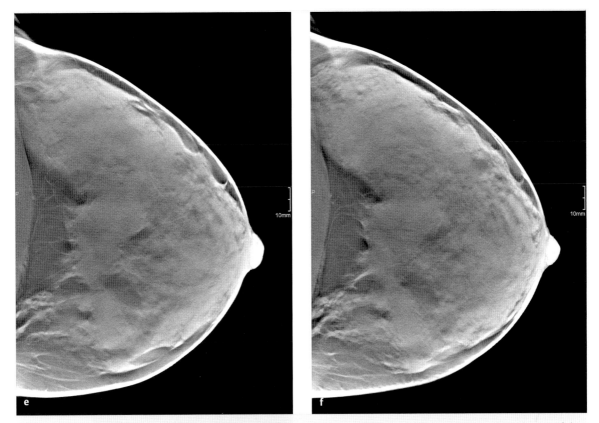

Fig. 5.27 (continued) Case 27. Screening examination of a 48-year-old woman. **(e)** Single slice from 3D tomosynthesis data set of the left breast, CC projection. Microcalcifications. **(f)** Single slice from 3D tomosynthesis data set of the left breast, CC projection. Microcalcifications.

5.2.28 Case 28

History

Patient is a nulliparous with no family history of breast cancer. No hormone therapy or prior breast surgery. She complains of pain in both breasts, more severe on the right, 1 month after trauma to the chest. No palpable breast masses or enlarged locoregional lymph nodes.

Mammography

Right breast: ACR 3. No suspicious masses or microcalcifications. BI-RADS 1 (**Fig. 5.28a, c**). Left breast: ACR 3. Mass with ill-defined margins in the lower inner quadrant, with faint microcalcifications. Classified as BI-RADS 4 (**Fig. 5.28b, d**).

DBT

MLO view of the left breast shows a lobulated mass measuring 9 × 4 mm in the lower inner quadrant, with partially indistinct margins and associated microcalcifications (**Fig. 5.28e, f, Video 5.15**).

Ultrasonography

No definite evidence of a mass.

Further Case History

Stereotactically guided vacuum biopsy indicated DCIS. Lesion was classified as B5a.

Final Diagnosis

DCIS.

Discussion

The margins of the mass in the lower inner quadrant of the left breast are displayed much more clearly by tomosynthesis than by conventional mammography. Also, the microcalcifications in the lesion are defined at least as well by tomosynthesis as by conventional mammography.

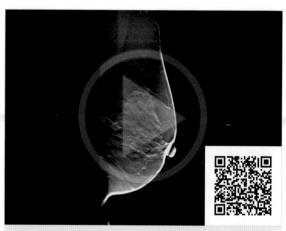

Video 5.15 Case 28. DBT data set of the left breast, MLO projection. A lobulated mass of 9 × 4 mm with partially indistinct margins and microcalcifications is detected in the lower inner quadrant.

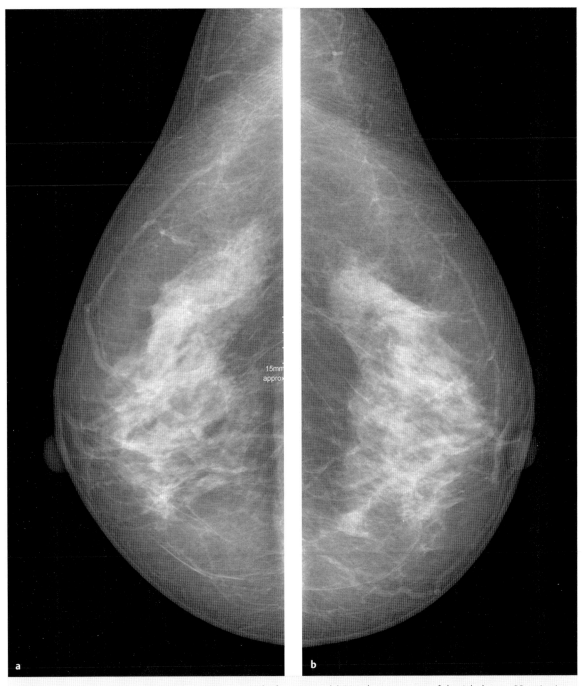

15mm
approx

a

b

Fig. 5.28 Case 28. Patient with bilateral breast pain 1 month after trauma. **(a)** Digital mammogram of the right breast, CC projection. **(b)** Digital mammogram of the left breast, CC projection.

continued ▶

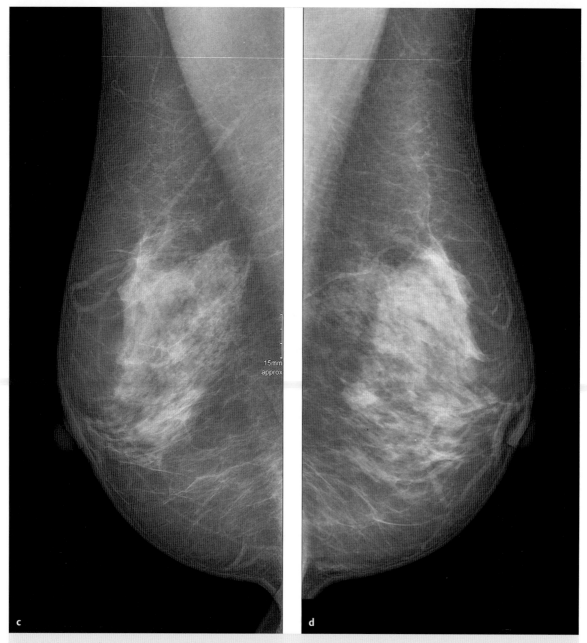

15mm
approx

c

d

Fig. 5.28 (continued) Case 28. Patient with bilateral breast pain 1 month after trauma. **(c)** Digital mammogram of the right breast, MLO projection. **(d)** Digital mammogram of the left breast, MLO projection.

continued ▶

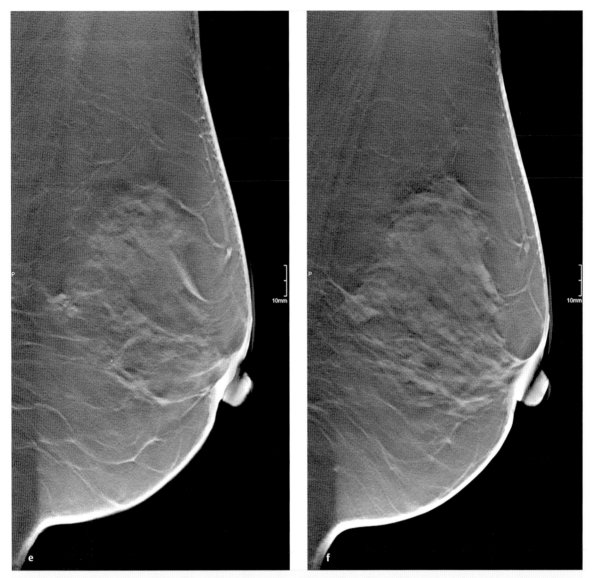

Fig. 5.28 (continued) Case 28. Patient with bilateral breast pain 1 month after trauma. **(e)** Single slice from 3D tomosynthesis data set of the left breast, MLO projection. Mass. **(f)** Single slice from 3D tomosynthesis data set of the left breast, MLO projection. Mass.

5.2.29 Case 29

History

Woman 55 years of age, a nulliparous, 5 years after BCS for invasive carcinoma NST of the left breast. Tumor stage T 1 a N0 M0. She presents now for follow-up.

Mammography

Right breast: ACR 3. Nodular pattern of fibrocystic changes with multiple rounded, monomorphic microcalcifications. Some of the calcifications are relatively coarse and have a "tea cup" appearance toward the center of the breast. MLO projection shows architectural distortion in the upper portion of the breast parenchyma, 5 cm from the nipple (**Fig. 5.29c**). This distortion is not visible in the CC projection (**Fig. 5.29a**). Classified as BI-RADS 4a. Left breast: ACR 3. Unchanged scar with architectural distortion in the upper outer quadrant, with rounded, monomorphic microcalcifications and central areas of liponecrosis. Classified as BI-RADS 2 (**Fig. 5.29b, d**).

DBT

DBT of the right breast in the CC and MLO projections. Both views demonstrate a 4-mm spiculated lesion in the upper outer quadrant, 5 cm from the nipple. The rounded, evenly spaced microcalcifications, some with a "tea cup" appearance, are clearly depicted, along with fibrocystic parenchymal changes. Classified as BI-RADS 4b (**Fig. 5.29e–h**).

Ultrasonography

Ultrasonography does not show a correlate for the mammographic findings.

Further Case History

Stereotactic vacuum biopsy indicated a radial scar and an associated 2-mm focus of invasive carcinoma NST.

Final Diagnosis

Radial scar and associated carcinoma (pT 1 a N0 M0).

Discussion

The spiculated lesion is faintly visible in just one mammographic view and cannot be positively distinguished from a summation artifact, whereas the lesion is clearly visualized in both tomosynthesis views. One-view tomosynthesis would have been sufficient in this case to confirm the lesion. Owing to radiation safety concerns, it is generally good practice to limit initial tomosynthesis to one view, as this will be sufficient to identify most mammographically indeterminate lesions. More studies are needed to determine whether, and in what cases, two-view tomosynthesis can add relevant diagnostic information.

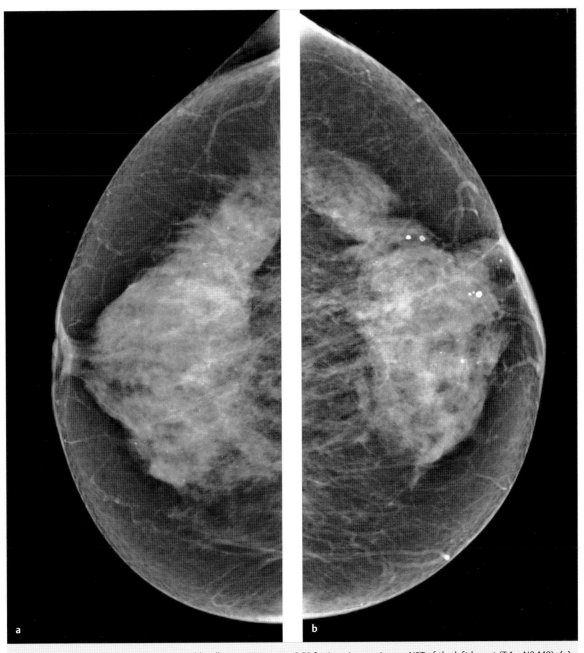

Fig. 5.29 Case 29. Follow-up of a 55-year-old nullipara, status post-BCS for invasive carcinoma NST of the left breast (T 1 a N0 M0). **(a)** Digital mammogram of the right breast, CC projection. **(b)** Digital mammogram of the left breast, CC projection.

continued ▶

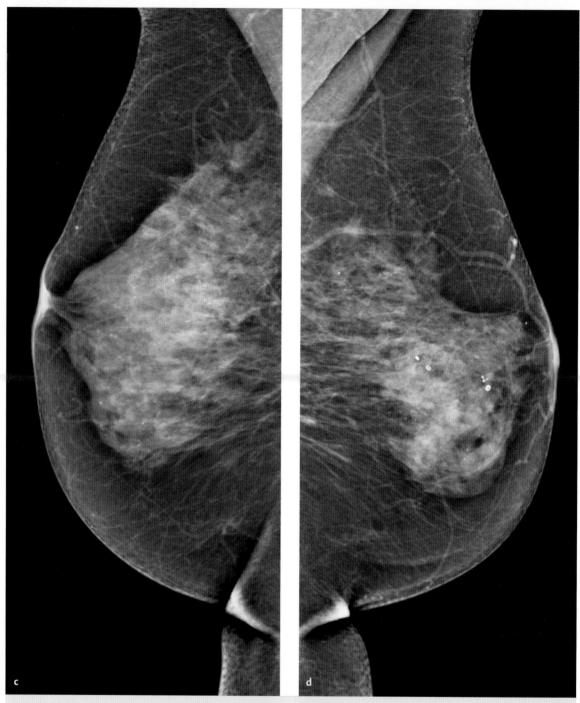

Fig. 5.29 (continued) Case 29. Follow-up of a 55-year-old nullipara, status post-BCS for invasive carcinoma NST of the left breast (T 1 a N0 M0). **(c)** Digital mammogram of the right breast, MLO projection. **(d)** Digital mammogram of the left breast, MLO projection.

continued ▶

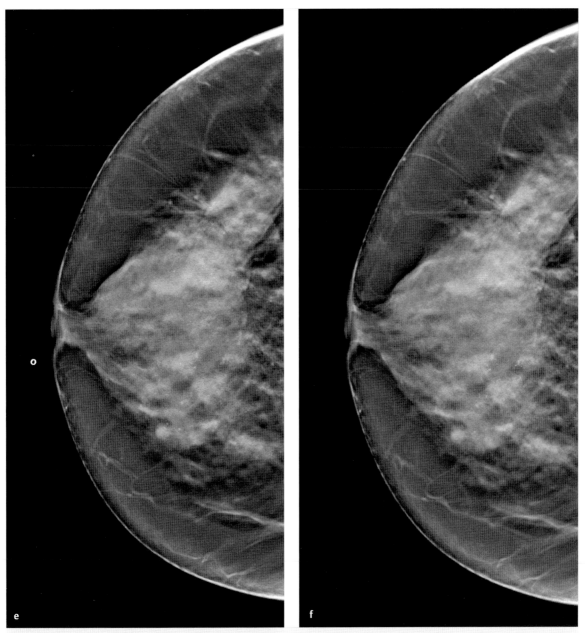

Fig. 5.29 (continued) Case 29. Follow-up of a 55-year-old nullipara, status post-BCS for invasive carcinoma NST of the left breast (T 1 a N0 M0). **(e)** Single slice from 3D tomosynthesis data set of the right breast, CC projection. **(f)** Adjacent slice from the same data set, CC projection.

continued ▶

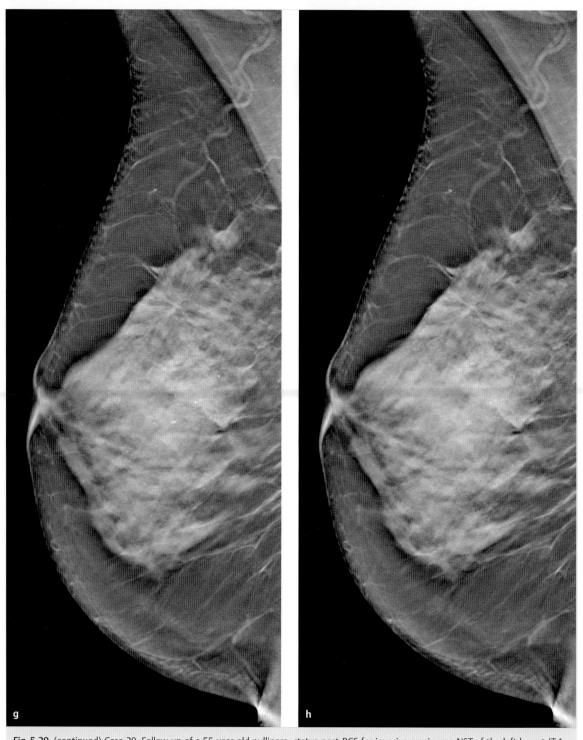

g

h

Fig. 5.29 (continued) Case 29. Follow-up of a 55-year-old nullipara, status post-BCS for invasive carcinoma NST of the left breast (T 1 a N0 M0). (g) Single slice from 3D tomosynthesis data set of the right breast, MLO projection. (h) Adjacent slice from the same data set, MLO projection.

5.2.30 Case 30

History

Woman 71 years of age with a maternal history of breast cancer before menopause. The patient is asymptomatic and has no visible or palpable abnormalities in either breast.

Mammography

Right breast: ACR 3. Vascular calcification with no suspicious microcalcifications and no masses. Nonspecific axillary lymph nodes. Classified as BI-RADS 2 (**Fig. 5.30a, c**). Left breast: ACR 3. Coarse, rounded calcifications at the center of the breast. Nonspecific axillary lymph nodes (**Fig. 5.30d**). CC view shows a density measuring 8 × 7 mm, located 2.5 cm behind the nipple (**Fig. 5.30b**); this area is new relative to prior mammograms (**Fig. 5.30e, f**). The finding is classified as BI-RADS 4.

Spot Compression View

Spot compression view of the left breast in the CC projection. The subareolar density is not definitely reproduced in this view (**Fig. 5.30 g**).

DBT

DBT of the left breast in the CC projection does not demonstrate a mass. The mammographic density is identified by tomosynthesis as a summation artifact, and is reclassified as BI-RADS 2 (**Fig. 5.30h, i**).

Final Diagnosis

Retroareolar summation artifact in the left breast. Both breasts classified as BI-RADS 2.

Discussion

The suspicious mammographic finding in this case is correctly characterized by both tomosynthesis and spot compression mammography. In large studies on this topic, tomosynthesis was found to be superior to spot compression views. Thus, tomosynthesis may be considered the imaging study of first choice for the further investigation of indeterminate mammographic findings.

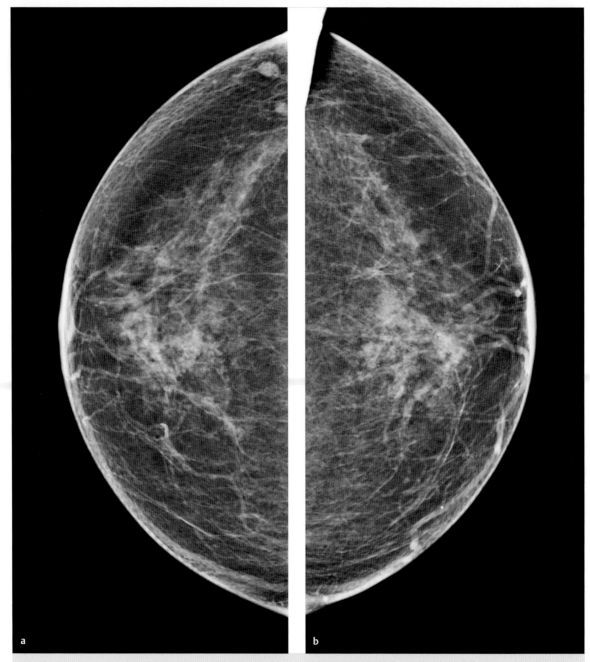

Fig. 5.30 Case 30. Screening examination of a 71-year-old woman. **(a)** Digital mammogram of the right breast, CC projection. **(b)** Digital mammogram of the left breast, CC projection.

continued ▶

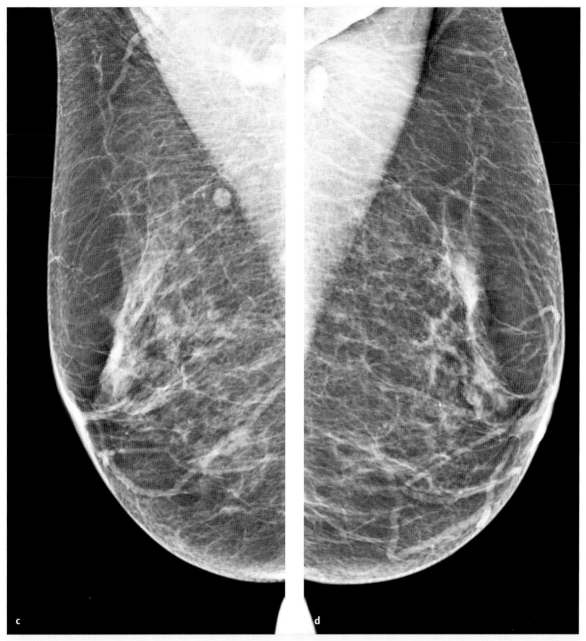

Fig. 5.30 (continued) Case 30. Screening examination of a 71-year-old woman. **(c)** Digital mammogram of the right breast, MLO projection. **(d)** Digital mammogram of the left breast, MLO projection.

continued ▶

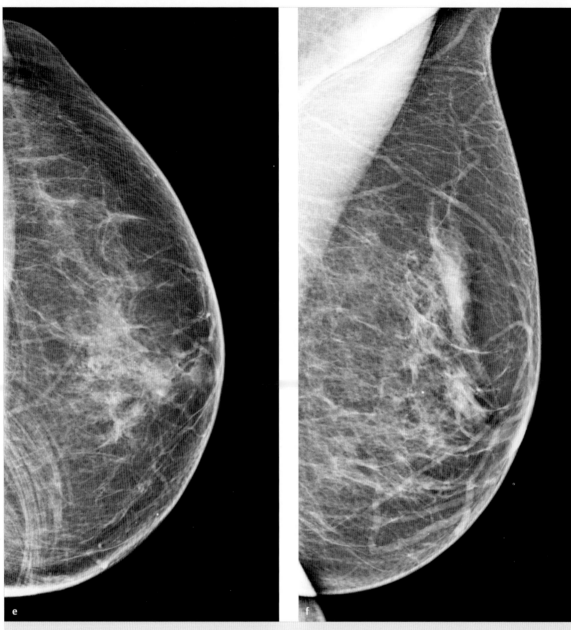

Fig. 5.30 (continued) Case 30. Screening examination of a 71-year-old woman. **(e)** Prior digital mammogram (18 months earlier) of the left breast, CC projection. **(f)** Prior digital mammogram (18 months earlier) of the left breast, MLO projection.

continued ▶

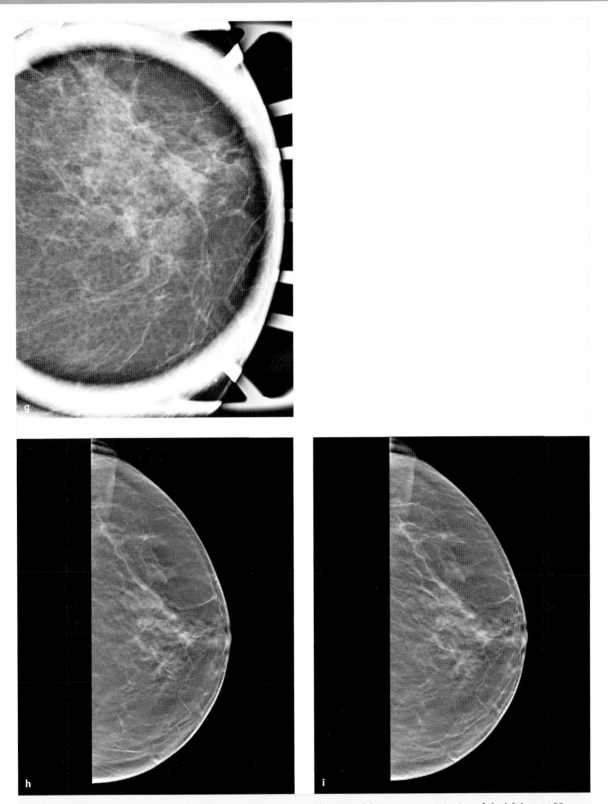

Fig. 5.30 (continued) Case 30. Screening examination of a 71-year-old woman. **(g)** Spot compression view of the left breast, CC projection. **(h)** Single slice from 3D tomosynthesis data set of the left breast, CC projection. **(i)** Single slice from 3D tomosynthesis data set of the left breast, CC projection.

5.2.31 Case 31

History

Woman 49 years of age has no family history of breast cancer and is not on hormone therapy. G3, P3. Status post-excisional biopsy of the right breast in 1994 with benign histology. No visible or palpable breast abnormalities.

Mammography

Right breast: ACR 3. No masses or microcalcifications. Classified as BI-RADS 2 (**Fig. 5.31a, c**). Left breast: ACR 3. A small mass is visible in the MLO view but does not appear in the CC view. Classified as BI-RADS 4 (**Fig. 5.31b, d**).

DBT

MLO view of the left breast demonstrates a 5-mm mass in the upper outer quadrant, 15 cm from the nipple. Owing to its irregular spiculated shape, the lesion is classified as BI-RADS 5 (**Fig. 5.31e, Video 5.16**).

MRI

Magnetic resonance (MR) mammography confirms an irregular mass in the upper outer quadrant of the left breast. The lesion shows early contrast enhancement (**Fig. 5.31f**).

Ultrasonography

Ultrasonography does not show a correlate for the mass detected by radiography and MRI.

Further Case History

MR-guided core-needle biopsy identified the lesion as moderately differentiated invasive carcinoma NST.

Final Diagnosis

Moderately differentiated invasive carcinoma NST 10 mm in diameter.

Discussion

The spiculated density in the upper outer quadrant of the left breast is more accurately displayed and characterized by tomosynthesis than by mammography. Because there was no sonographic correlate and stereotactic localization was imprecise, the lesion was investigated further by MRI. Tomosynthesis-guided biopsy would have been helpful in this case but was not available at the time of the examination.

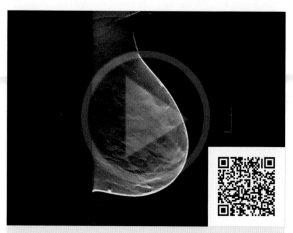

Video 5.16 Case 31. DBT data set of the left breast, MLO projection, shows a 0.5-cm mass in the upper outer quadrant, 15 cm from the nipple. Note the irregular, spiculated margins.

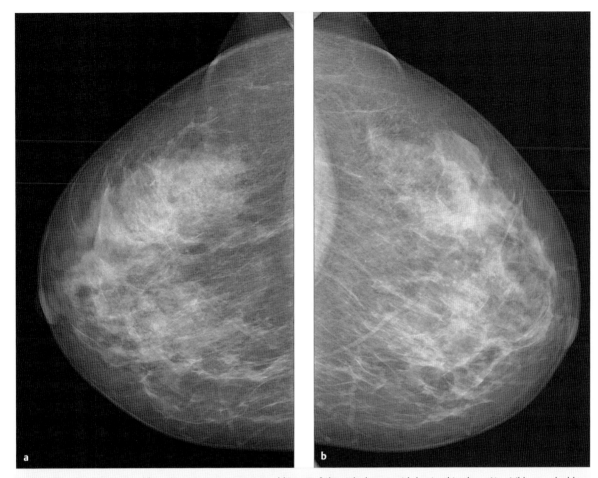

Fig. 5.31 Case 31. 49-year-old woman, status post-excisional biopsy of the right breast with benign histology. No visible or palpable abnormalities. **(a)** Digital mammogram of the right breast, CC projection. **(b)** Digital mammogram of the left breast, CC projection.

continued ▶

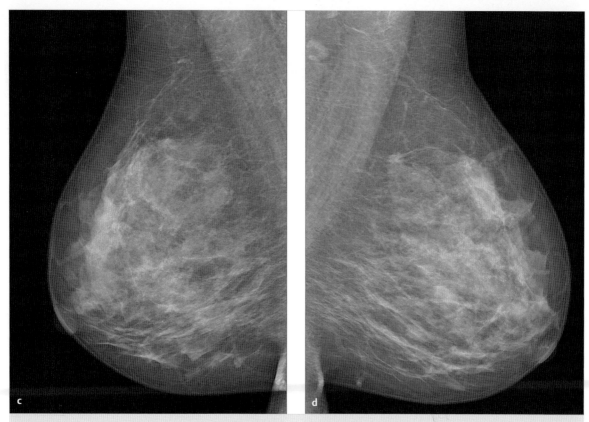

Fig. 5.31 (continued) Case 31. 49-year-old woman, status post-excisional biopsy of the right breast with benign histology. No visible or palpable abnormalities. **(c)** Digital mammogram of the right breast, MLO projection. **(d)** Digital mammogram of the left breast, MLO projection.

continued ▶

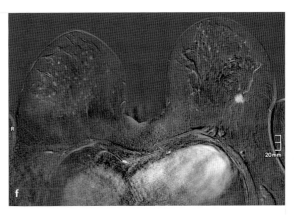

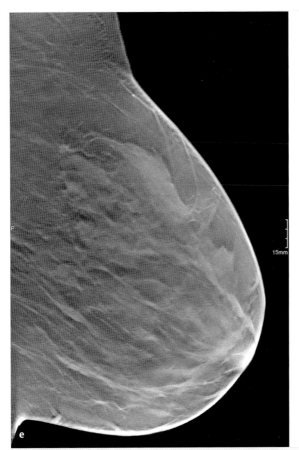

Fig. 5.31 (continued) Case 31. 49-year-old woman, status post-excisional biopsy of the right breast with benign histology. No visible or palpable abnormalities. (e) Single slice from 3D tomosynthesis data set of the left breast, MLO projection. Mass. (f) MR subtraction image 2 minutes after contrast administration.

5.2.32 Case 32

History

Woman 48 years of age, no family history of breast cancer, not on hormone therapy. G2, P2, breastfed for 9 and 10 months. The patient felt a nodule at the 2 o'clock position in her right breast.

Mammography

Right breast: ACR 4. Architectural distortion at the 3 o'clock position, classified as BI-RADS 4 (**Fig. 5.32a, b**). Left breast: ACR 4. No masses or microcalcifications, classified as BI-RADS 2.

Ultrasonography

Hypoechoic mass with ill-defined margins at the 2 o'clock position, measuring 1.7 × 1.3 × 1.8 cm (**Fig. 5.32c**), investigated by ultrasound-guided core-needle biopsy.

DBT

MLO view of the right breast shows air inclusions in the upper prepectoral region after core biopsy. A 0.7-cm spiculated mass is visible directly adjacent to that site (**Fig. 5.32 d, Video 5.17**).

Further Case History

DBT after ultrasound-guided core-needle biopsy confirmed the mass and air inclusions, thus providing correlation with the sonographic and mammographic findings. Histology showed only tumor-free breast tissue. Because core-needle histology did not adequately explain the spiculated lesion, a definitive diagnosis was established by wire localization and excisional biopsy.

Final Diagnosis

Fibrocystic changes with ductal epithelial hyperplasia and sclerosing adenosis. No evidence of a radial scar or malignancy.

Discussion

The high sensitivity of tomosynthesis in detecting architectural distortion leads to a higher false-positive rate. While DBT detected significantly more breast masses in all large clinical studies, its specificity was slightly below that of mammography in some cases.[1]

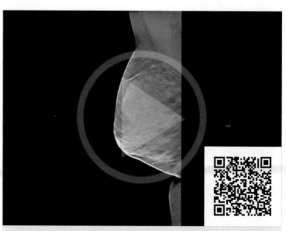

Video 5.17 Case 32. DBT data set of the right breast, MLO projection.

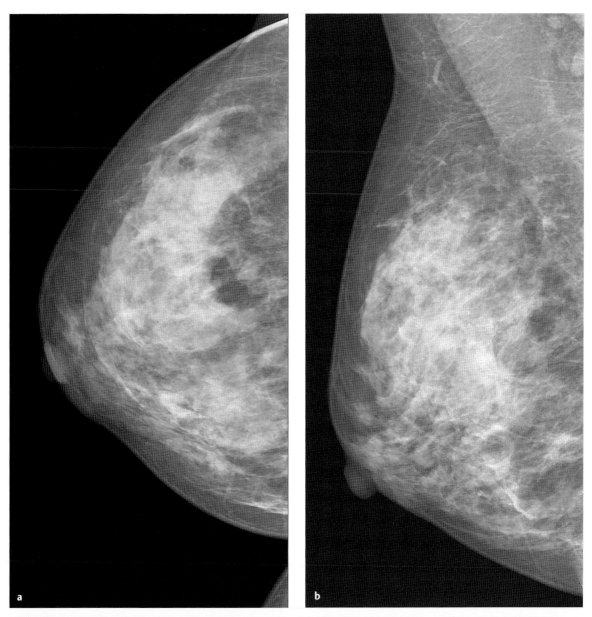

Fig. 5.32 Case 32. 48-year-old woman with a right breast nodule at the 2 o'clock position found on self-examination. **(a)** Digital mammogram of the right breast, CC projection. **(b)** Digital mammogram of the right breast, MLO projection.

continued ▶

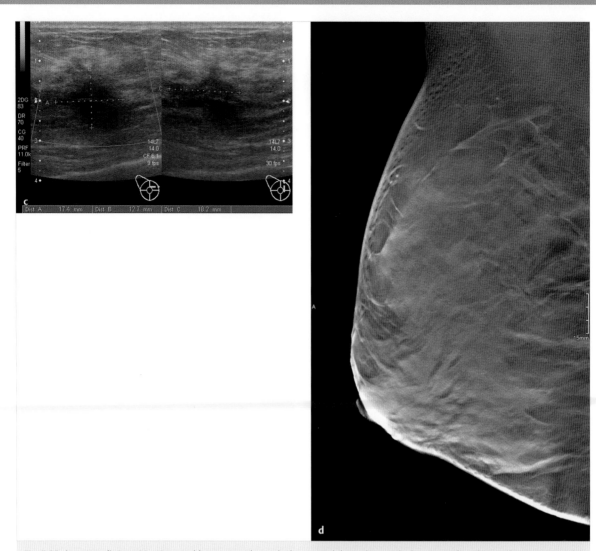

Fig. 5.32 (continued) Case 32. 48-year-old woman with a right breast nodule at the 2 o'clock position found on self-examination. **(c)** Ultrasound scan of the mass. **(d)** Single slice from 3D tomosynthesis data set of the right breast, MLO projection.

5.2.33 Case 33

History

Woman 67 years of age underwent a left mastectomy in 1993 for invasive carcinoma NST (pT 1 c pN0 M0), with no adjuvant therapy. Seen at follow-up, she has a well-healed chest wall scar on the left side with no palpable abnormalities. The right breast is clinically normal and there is no evidence of enlarged axillary nodes on either side.

Mammography

Right breast: ACR 3. Moderately coarse pattern of fibrocystic changes with microcalcifications and vascular calcification. Solitary, round microcalcifications; none appear suspicious. MLO view shows a density with ill-defined margins in the upper portion of the breast, approximately 7.5 cm from the nipple (**Fig. 5.33b**). No definite correlate in the CC view (**Fig. 5.33a**). Classified as BI-RADS 4b. The density was not yet visible in prior mammograms taken 1 year earlier (**Fig. 5.33c, d**).

DBT

CC and MLO views of the right breast clearly demonstrate a 4-mm spiculated mass at the 11 o'clock position in the upper outer quadrant, 7 cm from the nipple. Classified as BI-RADS 5 (**Fig. 5.33e, f**).

Ultrasonography

Ultrasound scan of the right breast shows a hypoechoic, vertically oriented oval mass with ill-defined margins at the 11 o'clock position, 6 cm from the nipple. It has a hyperechoic rim and posterior acoustic shadow. Dimensions 6 × 4 × 4 mm, classified as BI-RADS 5 (**Fig. 5.33g, h**).

Further Case History

Ultrasound-guided core-needle biopsy confirmed grade 2 invasive carcinoma NST.

Final Diagnosis

Invasive carcinoma NST.

Discussion

The small mass, visible in just one mammographic view, is clearly displayed in both tomosynthesis views as a spiculated lesion with ill-defined margins. One tomosynthesis view in either projection would have been sufficient in the present case. Very few data have been published, however, comparing the diagnostic accuracy of one-view and two-view DBT. Based on the 3D information and good clinical results obtained with one view, it does not appear necessary at present to perform tomosynthesis routinely in two projections.

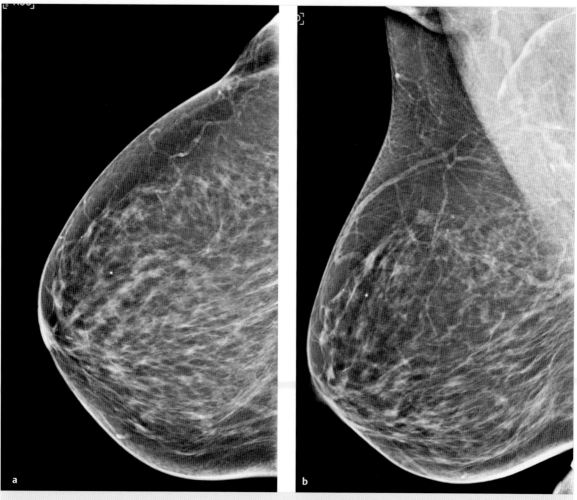

Fig. 5.33 Case 33. Follow-up of a 67-year-old woman, status post-left mastectomy for invasive carcinoma NST (pT 1 c pN0 M0). No adjuvant therapy. **(a)** Digital mammogram of the right breast, CC projection. **(b)** Digital mammogram of the right breast, MLO projection.

continued ▶

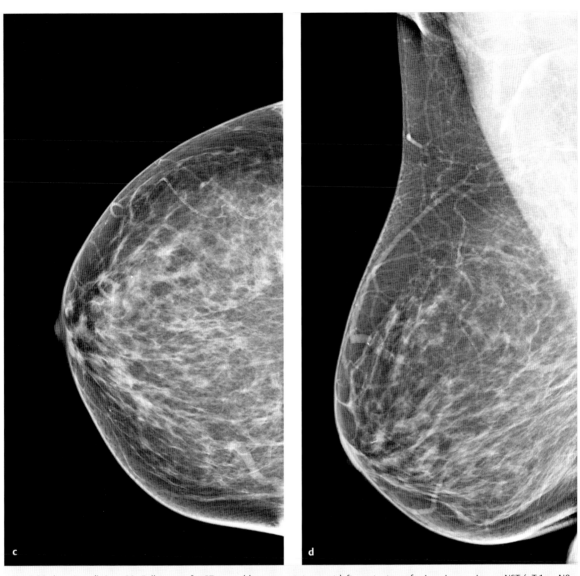

Fig. 5.33 (continued) Case 33. Follow-up of a 67-year-old woman, status post-left mastectomy for invasive carcinoma NST (pT 1 c pN0 M0). No adjuvant therapy. **(c)** Prior digital mammogram (1 year earlier) of the right breast, CC projection. **(d)** Prior digital mammogram (1 year earlier) of the right breast, MLO projection.

continued ▶

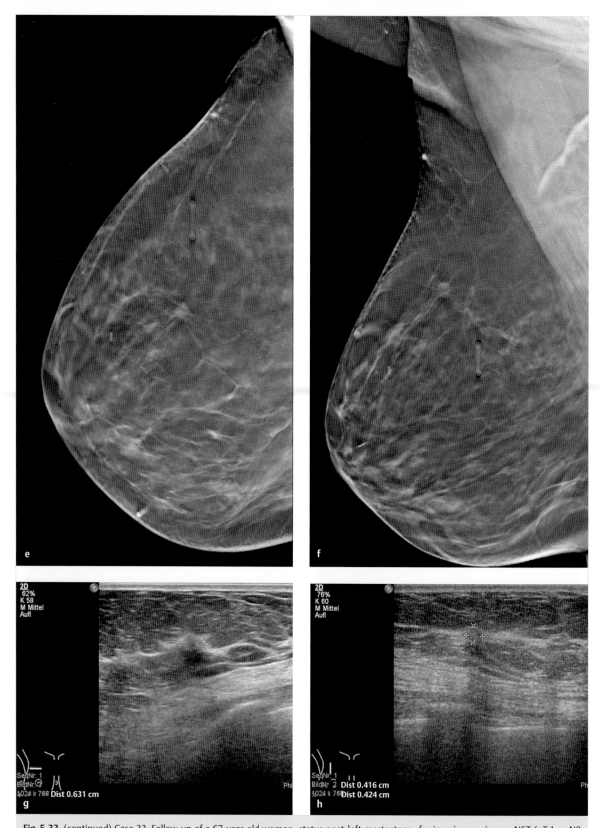

Fig. 5.33 (continued) Case 33. Follow-up of a 67-year-old woman, status post-left mastectomy for invasive carcinoma NST (pT 1 c pN0 M0). No adjuvant therapy. **(e)** Single slice from 3D tomosynthesis data set of the right breast, CC projection. **(f)** Single slice from 3D tomosynthesis data set of the right breast, MLO projection. **(g)** Ultrasound scan of the mass. **(h)** Ultrasound scan of the mass, second plane.

5.2.34 Case 34

History

Asymptomatic 59-year-old woman had a grandmother who developed breast cancer after menopause and a maternal cousin who was diagnosed in perimenopause. The patient has palpable fibrocystic nodules in both breasts. Axillary lymph nodes are not palpable on either side.

Mammography

Both breasts are ACR 3. Bilateral mammograms in the CC projection show a nodular to moderately coarse pattern of fibrocystic changes in both breasts. There are scattered, rounded, monomorphic microcalcifications and vascular calcifications but no suspicious microcalcifications or focal lesions. Both breasts classified as BI-RADS 2. Findings in the radiographically dense breasts are unchanged relative to prior mammograms (**Fig. 5.34a–f**).

DBT

MLO views of both breasts do not detect any masses or suspicious microcalcifications. Bilateral, nonspecific lymph nodes up to 1 cm in diameter are found in the axillary tail. Both breasts classified as BI-RADS 2 (**Fig. 5.34g, h**).

Final Diagnosis

Bilateral fibrocystic changes, BI-RADS 2.

Discussion

In this patient with radiographically dense breasts (ACR 3), one-view mammography (CC) was combined with complementary-view tomosynthesis (MLO), to permit a nonsuperimposed evaluation of the breast parenchyma. A recent study showed that lesions obscured by overlapping breast tissue were responsible for 81% of cancers not detected at mammography.[2] This suggests that the use of tomosynthesis may eliminate the most frequent cause of false-negative mammograms.

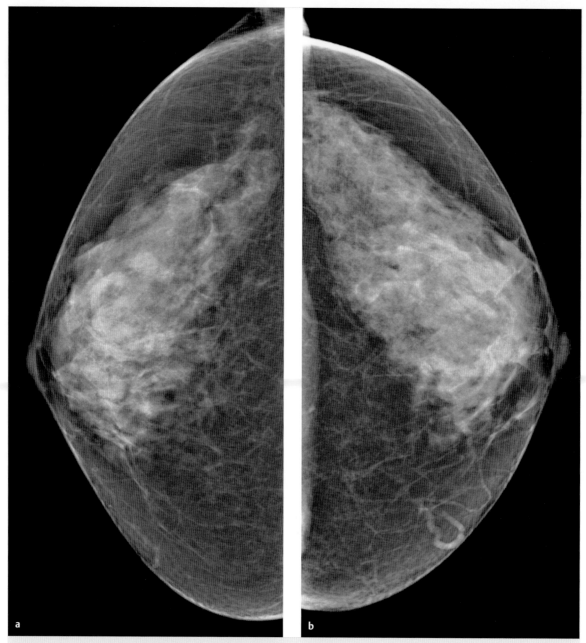

Fig. 5.34 Case 34. Screening examination of an asymptomatic 59-year-old woman with palpable fibrocystic nodules in both breasts. **(a)** Digital mammogram of the right breast, CC projection. **(b)** Digital mammogram of the left breast, CC projection. ACR 3.

continued ▶

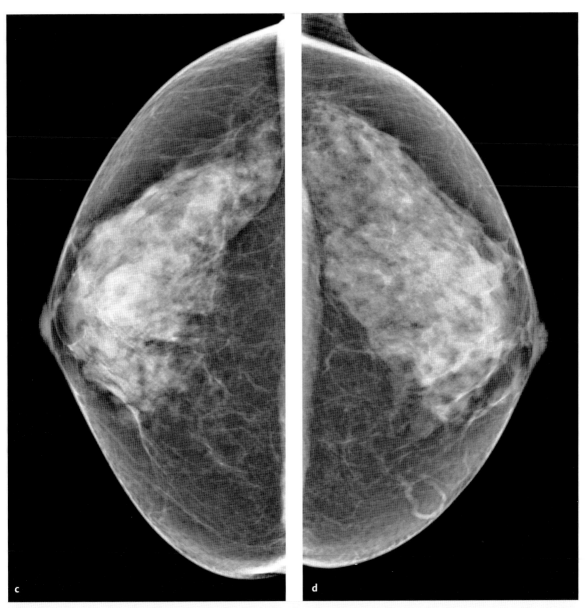

Fig. 5.34 (continued) Case 34. Screening examination of an asymptomatic 59-year-old woman with palpable fibrocystic nodules in both breasts. **(c)** Prior digital mammogram (1 year earlier) of the right breast, CC projection. **(d)** Prior digital mammogram (1 year earlier) of the left breast, CC projection.

continued ▶

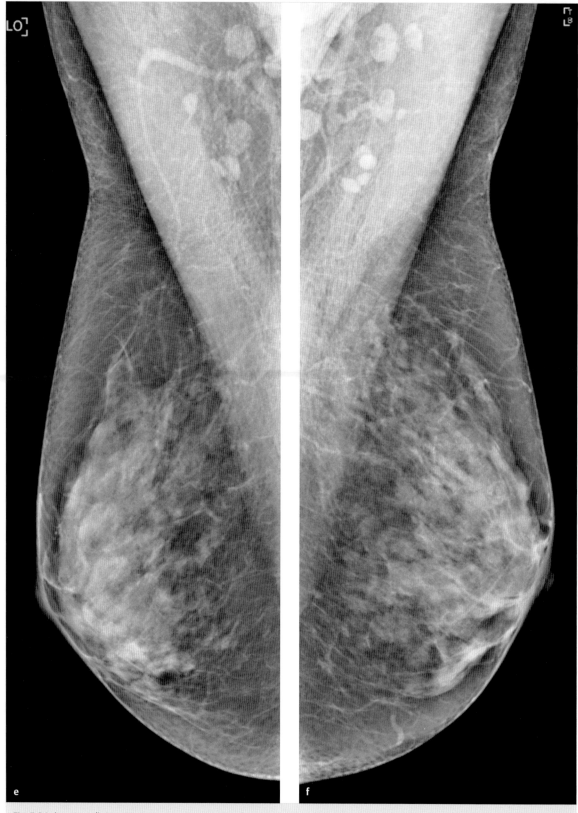

Fig. 5.34 (continued) Case 34. Screening examination of an asymptomatic 59-year-old woman with palpable fibrocystic nodules in both breasts. **(e)** Prior digital mammogram (1 year earlier) of the right breast, MLO projection. **(f)** Prior digital mammogram (1 year earlier) of the right breast, MLO projection.

continued ▶

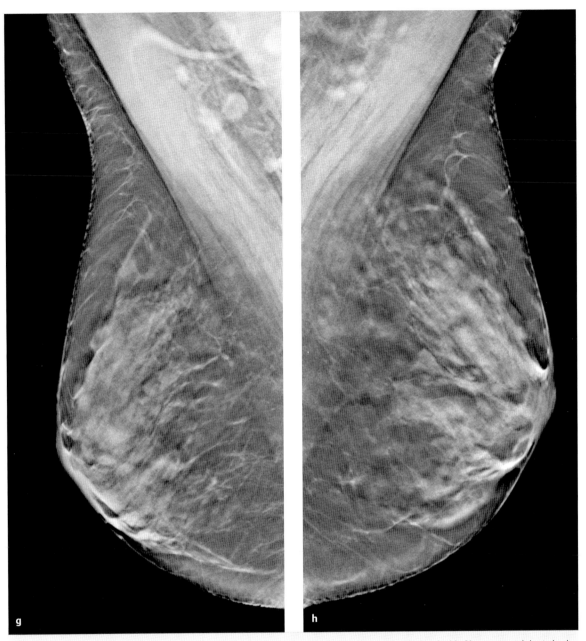

Fig. 5.34 (continued) Case 34. Screening examination of an asymptomatic 59-year-old woman with palpable fibrocystic nodules in both breasts. **(g)** Single slice from 3D tomosynthesis data set of the right breast, MLO projection. **(h)** Single slice from 3D tomosynthesis data set of the left breast, MLO projection.

5.2.35 Case 35

History

Woman 40 years of age. G2, P2, breastfed both children for 6 months. She has bilateral palpable, movable nodules and bilateral mastodynia. Her mother was diagnosed with breast cancer at age 48 years.

Mammography

Right breast: ACR 2. Multiple well-circumscribed masses of varying sizes. No suspicious masses or suspicious microcalcifications. Classified as BI-RADS 2 (**Fig. 5.35a, c**). Left breast: ACR 2. MLO mammogram shows a subtle spiculated density approximately 6 cm behind the nipple that does not have a definite correlate in the CC view. Multiple, predominantly monomorphic microcalcifications. Classified as BI-RADS 4 (**Fig. 5.35b, d**).

DBT

MLO view of the left breast shows a density of approximately 1.5 × 1.0 cm, with radiating spicules, surrounded by multiple monomorphic microcalcifications. Classified as BI-RADS 4 (**Fig. 5.35e, Video 5.18**).

Ultrasonography

Right breast: multiple cysts, no suspicious mass. Left breast: inhomogeneous hypoechoic area in the outer midbreast with adjacent aggregated cysts (**Fig. 5.35f**).

Further Case History

Ultrasound-guided core-needle biopsy of the left breast yielded tumor-free breast tissue with fibrocystic changes. Classified as B2. Based on the suspicious ultrasonography and tomosynthesis findings, it was decided to proceed with wire localization and local excision.

Final Diagnosis

Radial scar, B3 lesion.

Discussion

The spiculated mass is defined much more clearly by tomosynthesis than conventional mammography. In this case, tomosynthesis facilitates lesion detection and localization but does not increase the specificity of the mammographic diagnosis.

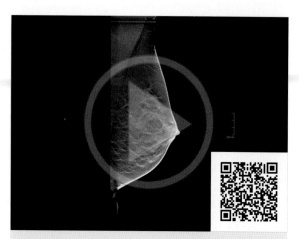

Video 5.18 Case 35. DBT data set of the left breast, MLO projection, shows a density measuring 1.5 × 1.0 cm, with radiating spicules, surrounded by multiple monomorphic microcalcifications.

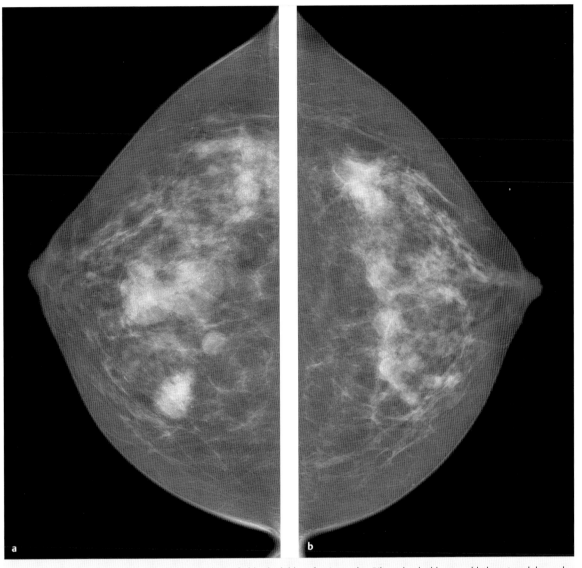

Fig. 5.35 Case 35. 40-year-old woman. G2, P2, breastfed both children for 6 months. Bilateral palpable, movable breast nodules and bilateral mastodynia. Family history of breast cancer. (a) Digital mammogram of the right breast, CC projection. (b) Digital mammogram of the left breast, CC projection.

continued ▶

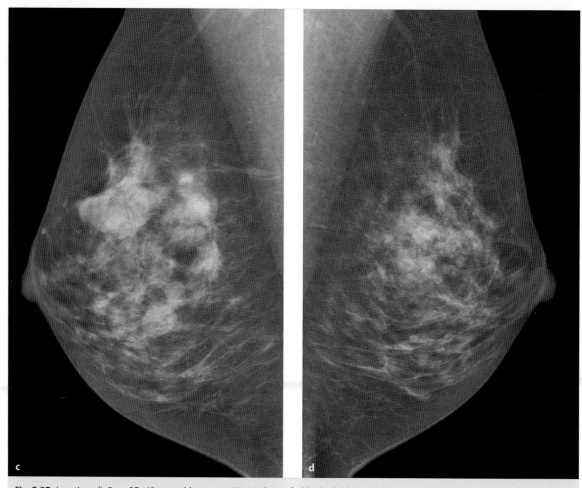

c

d

Fig. 5.35 (continued) Case 35. 40-year-old woman. G2, P2, breastfed both children for 6 months. Bilateral palpable, movable breast nodules and bilateral mastodynia. Family history of breast cancer. **(c)** Digital mammogram of the right breast, MLO projection. **(d)** Digital mammogram of the left breast, MLO projection.

continued ▶

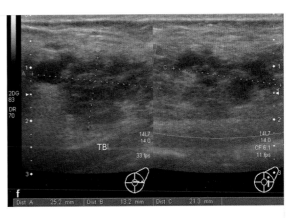

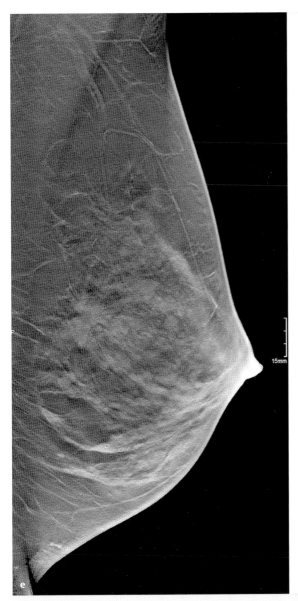

Fig. 5.35 (continued) Case 35. 40-year-old woman. G2, P2, breastfed both children for 6 months. Bilateral palpable, movable breast nodules and bilateral mastodynia. Family history of breast cancer. (e) Single slice from 3D tomosynthesis data set of the left breast, MLO projection. Spiculated mass. (f) Ultrasound scan of the mass.

5.2.36 Case 36

History

Woman 75 years of age. G3, P3, breastfed each child for 8 months. No family history of breast cancer. On physical examination, a firm, immovable 2-cm mass is noted in the upper inner quadrant of the left breast. Suspicious level 1 lymph nodes are also palpable in the axilla.

Mammography

Left breast: ACR 2. A spiculated mass measuring 2.5 × 2.3 × 2.3 cm, with associated coarse calcifications, is visible in the upper inner quadrant. Located 5 cm lateral and apical to that mass are three additional masses (7 mm, 4 mm, 3 mm), which are partly obscured by superimposed parenchyma. The large mass is classified as BI-RADS 5, the other three as BI-RADS 4. Two suspicious axillary lymph nodes measure 17 × 8 mm and 8 × 6 mm (**Fig. 5.36a, b**).

DBT

DBT of the left breast in the CC and MLO projections. The spiculated mass, which measures 2.7 × 2.4 × 2.3 cm, is clearly visualized. It is classified as BI-RADS 5. The other three masses, which were partially obscured on mammograms, are found on tomosynthesis (CC view) to have smooth margins on all sides, enabling them to be classified as benign (**Fig. 5.36c–f**).

Ultrasonography

The spiculated mammographic lesion correlates with a hypoechoic mass that is 1.8 × 2.1 × 2.0 cm with ill-defined margins, at the 11 o'clock position in the upper inner quadrant of the left breast. The mass has a hyperechoic rim and inhomogeneous posterior shadow (**Fig. 5.36g**). The small mammographic lesions at nipple level in the outer part of the breast correlate with well-circumscribed echo-free and hypoechoic masses, which are interpreted as cysts (**Fig. 5.36h**). Ultrasonography also shows a suspicious left axillary lymph node, measuring 1.1 × 1.9 × 1.5 cm (**Fig. 5.36i**).

Further Case History

Ultrasound-guided core-needle biopsy identified the mass as grade 3 invasive carcinoma NST. The three small, hypoechoic masses were all investigated by fine-needle aspiration cytology and were identified as benign breast cysts.

Final Diagnosis

Solitary invasive carcinoma NST with axillary lymph node metastasis.

Discussion

The spiculated mass clearly meets the criteria for a BI-RADS 5 lesion on mammography, ultrasonography, and tomosynthesis, but tomosynthesis can provide nonsuperimposed views of the other three small masses in the upper outer quadrant of the left breast. Their smooth margins on tomosynthesis slices identify these lesions as breast cysts. In the present case, tomosynthesis alone supplies a level of information that only the combination of mammography plus ultrasonography can provide using standard techniques.

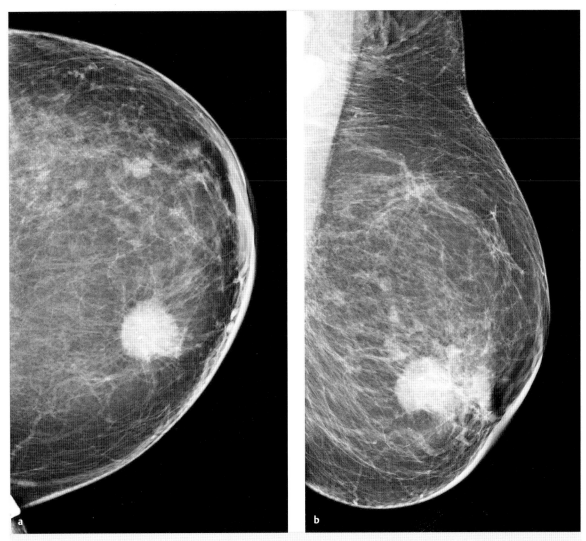

Fig. 5.36 Case 36. 75-year-old woman with a firm, immovable breast mass and suspicious, palpable level 1 axillary lymph nodes. **(a)** Digital mammogram of the left breast, CC projection. **(b)** Digital mammogram of the left breast, MLO projection.

continued ▶

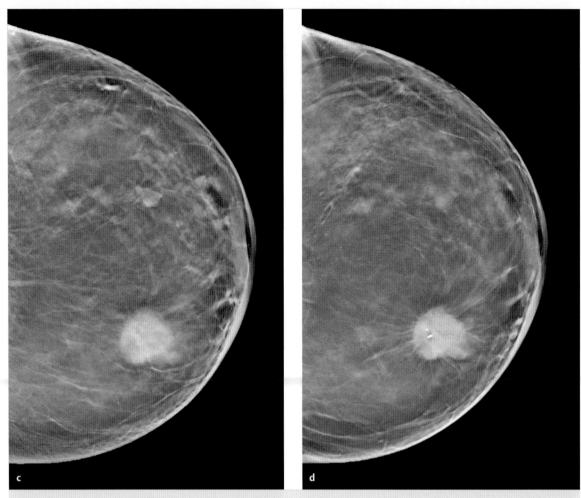

Fig. 5.36 (continued) Case 36. 75-year-old woman with a firm, immovable breast mass and suspicious, palpable level 1 axillary lymph nodes. **(c)** Single slice from 3D tomosynthesis data set of the left breast, CC projection. **(d)** Single slice from 3D tomosynthesis data set of the left breast, CC projection.

continued ▶

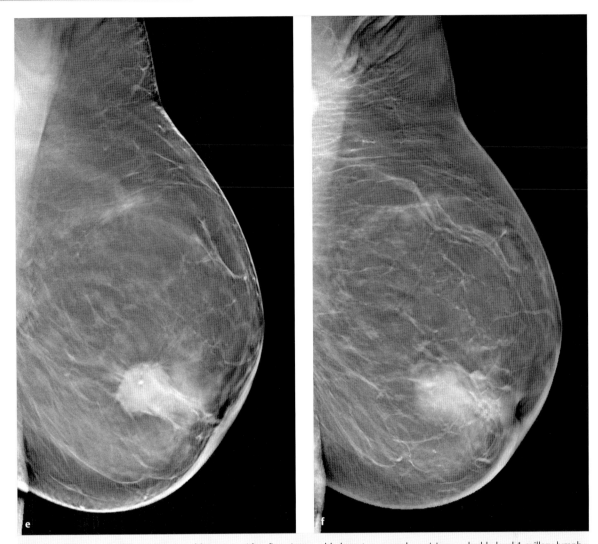

Fig. 5.36 (continued) Case 36. 75-year-old woman with a firm, immovable breast mass and suspicious, palpable level 1 axillary lymph nodes. (e) Single slice from 3D tomosynthesis data set of the left breast, MLO projection. (f) Single slice from 3D tomosynthesis data set of the left breast, MLO projection.

continued ▶

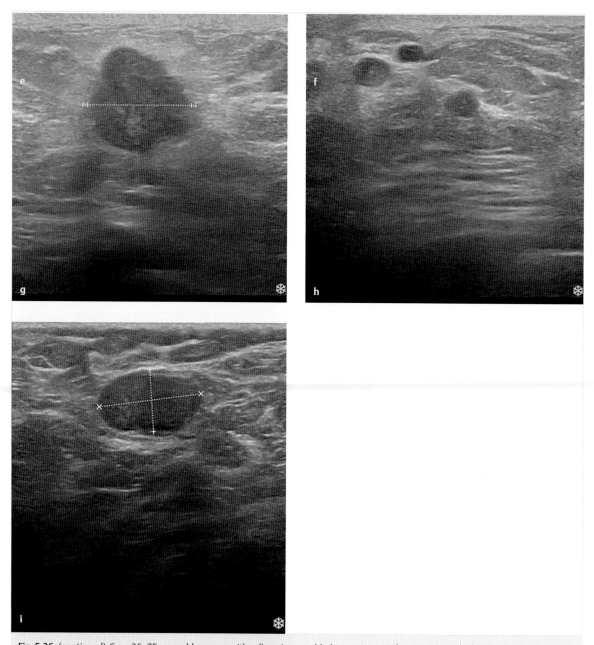

Fig. 5.36 (continued) Case 36. 75-year-old woman with a firm, immovable breast mass and suspicious, palpable level 1 axillary lymph nodes. **(g)** Ultrasound scan of the BI-RADS 5 lesion in the upper inner quadrant of the left breast. **(h)** Ultrasound scan of the three small masses in the upper outer quadrant. **(i)** Ultrasound scan of a suspicious left axillary lymph node, 1.1 × 1.9 × 1.5 cm.

5.2.37 Case 37

History

Woman 75 years of age, G2, P2. She has a family history of breast cancer (sister and aunt). Status post-bilateral open breast biopsies with benign histology. Surgical scars in the lateral periareolar area of the right breast and lower outer quadrant of the left breast appear well healed. No palpable masses or enlarged axillary nodes.

Mammography

Right breast: ACR 2. No masses. Two nonsuspicious microcalcifications are projected adjacent to each other in the upper outer quadrant (**Fig. 5.37a, c**). Left breast: ACR 2. An approximately 8-mm mass is visible in the upper breast in the MLO view. It does not have a definite correlate in the CC view. Flocculent, monomorphic microcalcifications are present approximately 3 cm behind the nipple, and a spindle-shaped opacity measuring approximately 2 × 1 cm is visible in the lower central breast (**Fig. 5.37b, d**). The mass in the MLO view is classified as BI-RADS 4.

DBT

MLO view of the left breast shows a spiculated mass with irregular margins in the upper outer quadrant (**Fig. 5.37e**), retroareolar monomorphic microcalcifications (**Fig. 5.37f**), and a well-circumscribed, elongated density in the lower central breast (**Fig. 5.37 g**). The lesion in the upper outer quadrant is classified as BI-RADS 5 (**Video 5.19**).

Ultrasonography

Inhomogeneous echo texture in the upper outer quadrant, 8 mm in diameter, may correspond to the mammographic mass. No other masses are seen (**Fig. 5.37h**).

MRI

An 8-mm mass in the upper outer quadrant shows intense, early enhancement on MRI. The elongated structure in the lower central breast does not enhance (**Fig. 5.37i, j**).

Further Case History

Stereotactic core-needle biopsy revealed invasive, moderately differentiated lobular carcinoma. The elongated density in the lower central breast, interpreted as a scar, and the microcalcification cluster were unchanged over a 2-year period.

Final Diagnosis

Invasive, moderately differentiated lobular carcinoma.

Discussion

This case illustrates the higher specificity of tomosynthesis compared with mammography. The carcinoma can be more accurately detected and characterized with DBT, as can the benign microcalcification cluster and the scar in the lower central breast.

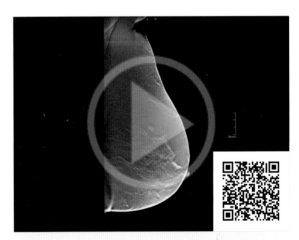

Video 5.19 Case 37. DBT data set of the left breast, MLO projection. Spiculated mass with irregular margins in the upper outer quadrant, retroareolar monomorphic microcalcifications, and an elongated density with smooth margins in the lower central breast.

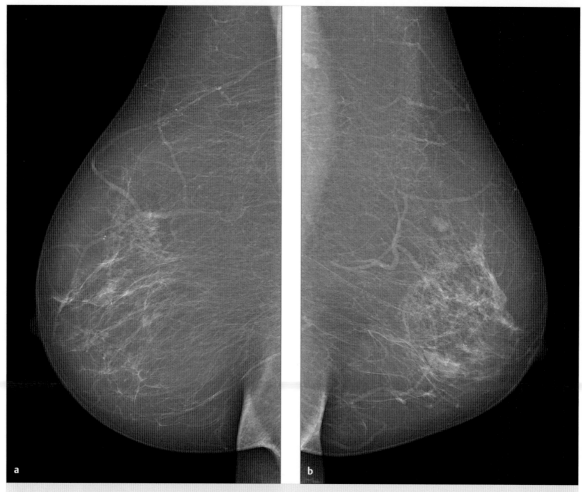

Fig. 5.37 Case 37. 75-year-old woman, status post-bilateral open breast biopsies with benign results. Well-healed scars, no palpable breast masses or enlarged axillary lymph nodes. **(a)** Digital mammogram of the right breast, MLO projection. **(b)** Digital mammogram of the left breast, MLO projection.

continued ▶

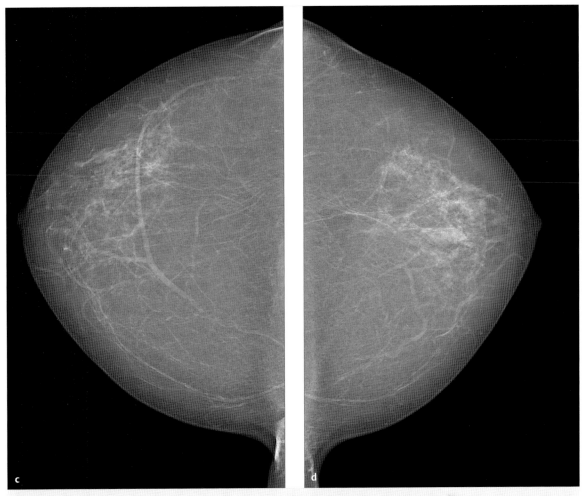

Fig. 5.37 (continued) Case 37. 75-year-old woman, status post-bilateral open breast biopsies with benign results. Well-healed scars, no palpable breast masses or enlarged axillary lymph nodes. (c) Digital mammogram of the right breast, CC projection. (d) Digital mammogram of the left breast, CC projection.

continued ▶

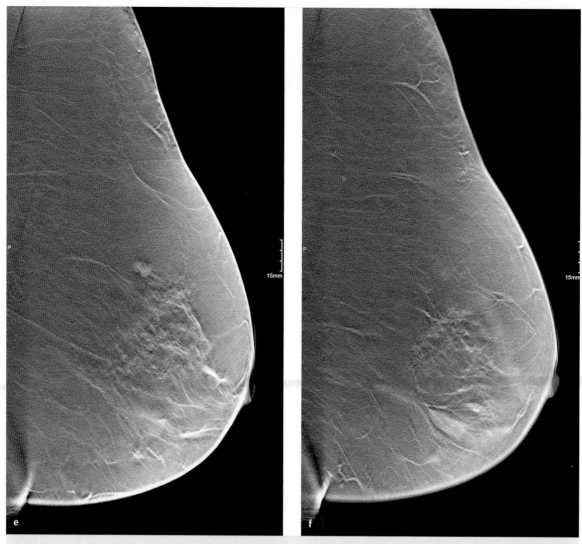

Fig. 5.37 (continued) Case 37. 75-year-old woman, status post-bilateral open breast biopsies with benign results. Well-healed scars, no palpable breast masses or enlarged axillary lymph nodes. **(e)** Single slice from 3D tomosynthesis data set of the left breast, MLO projection. Carcinoma. **(f)** Single slice from 3D tomosynthesis data set of the left breast, MLO projection. Microcalcification cluster.

continued ▶

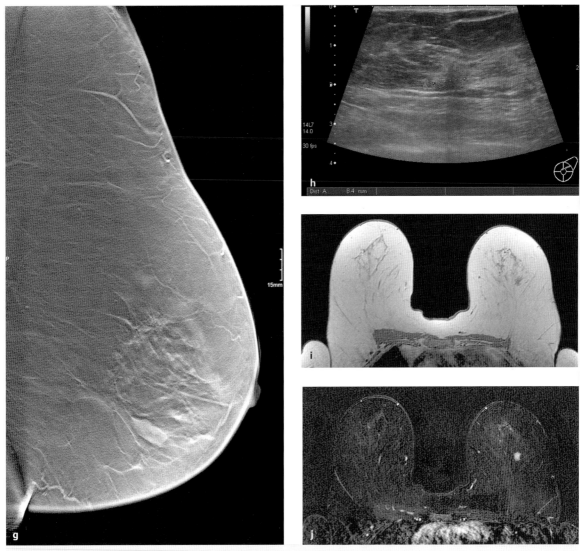

Fig. 5.37 (continued) Case 37. 75-year-old woman, status post-bilateral open breast biopsies with benign results. Well-healed scars, no palpable breast masses or enlarged axillary lymph nodes. **(g)** Single slice from 3D tomosynthesis data set of the left breast, MLO projection. Benign mass. **(h)** Ultrasound scan of the mass in the upper outer quadrant. **(i)** Unenhanced T 1-weighted MRI demonstrates an 8-mm mass in the left breast. **(j)** MR subtraction image of the left breast 1 minute after contrast administration.

5.2.38 Case 38

History

Asymptomatic 72-year-old woman, nulliparous, with a family history of breast cancer. She has no visible or palpable abnormalities in either breast.

Mammography

Right breast: ACR 1. No masses or suspicious microcalcifications. Classified as BI-RADS 2 (**Fig. 5.38a, c**). Left breast: ACR 1. MLO view shows a 2.5-cm retroareolar architectural distortion with no correlate in the CC view. Classified as BI-RADS 4 (**Fig. 5.38b, d**). Supplemental ML view (**Fig. 5.38e**) does not demonstrate the lesion.

Spot Compression View

Spot compression view of the left breast does not show a correlate for the questionable mass (**Fig. 5.38f**).

DBT

DBT of the left breast in the MLO projection. Supplemental 3D tomosynthesis clearly identifies the mass as a summation artifact caused by residual parenchyma and overlapping tissues. Reclassified as BI-RADS 2 (**Fig. 5.38g, h**).

Final Diagnosis

Retroareolar summation artifact in the left breast, BI-RADS 2.

Discussion

The architectural distortion visible in just one mammographic view is positively identified by tomosynthesis and additional views as a summation artifact. Tomosynthesis in this case is equivalent to special views, although current studies show that DBT is superior to special views in the investigation of equivocal mammographic findings.

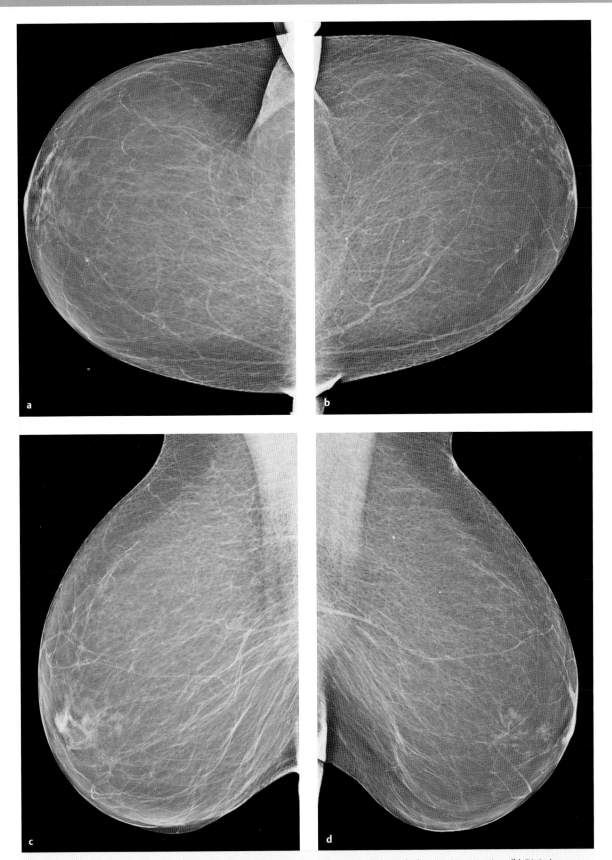

Fig. 5.38 Case 38. Asymptomatic 72-year-old woman. **(a)** Digital mammogram of the right breast, CC projection. **(b)** Digital mammogram of the left breast, CC projection. **(c)** Digital mammogram of the right breast, MLO projection. **(d)** Digital mammogram of the left breast, MLO projection.

continued ►

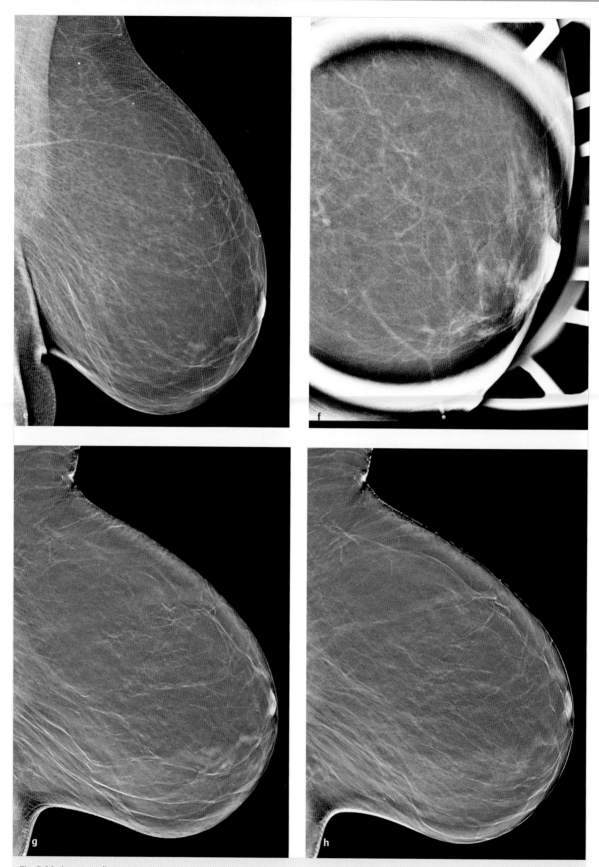

Fig. 5.38 (continued) Case 38. Asymptomatic 72-year-old woman. **(e)** Digital mammogram of the left breast, ML projection. **(f)** Spot compression view of the left breast, MLO projection. **(g)** Single slice from 3D tomosynthesis data set of the left breast, MLO projection. **(h)** Single slice from 3D tomosynthesis data set of the left breast, MLO projection.

5.2.39 Case 39

History

Woman 40 years of age, first diagnosed with multiple myeloma 5 years earlier. She was treated by high-dose chemotherapy and stem-cell transplantation. Intramammary involvement 2 years ago, treated by radiotherapy. She now has a 2-month history of bilateral, multiple, progressive palpable breast masses, approximately 1 cm in size. She has no family history of breast cancer.

Mammography

Right breast: ACR 3. Multiple masses up to 1 cm in size, partially obscured by superimposed parenchyma. Classified as BI-RADS 5 (**Fig. 5.39a**).

DBT

DBT of the right breast in the MLO projection. Tomosynthesis gives nonsuperimposed views of multiple, predominantly well-circumscribed lesions, up to 1 cm in size. Given the patient's history and multiple progressive findings, the lesions are classified as BI-RADS 5 (**Fig. 5.39b, c**).

Ultrasonography

Ultrasonography demonstrates multiple masses, some uniformly hypoechoic and some with echogenic centers. Scans show diffuse infiltration of the breast parenchyma (**Fig. 5.39d–g**), with profuse lesion blood flow (**Fig. 5.39i**). Static elastography shows areas of tissue hardening (**Fig. 5.39h**). Classified as BI-RADS 5.

Further Case History

Ultrasound-guided core-needle biopsy revealed new infiltration of the breast by known multiple myeloma.

Final Diagnosis

Multiple myeloma of the breast.

Discussion

Ultrasonography was definitely the most important imaging modality in this case, as it detected hyperperfusion and tissue hardening in masses that had a somewhat benign appearance on mammograms. Ultrasonography was also used for biopsy guidance.

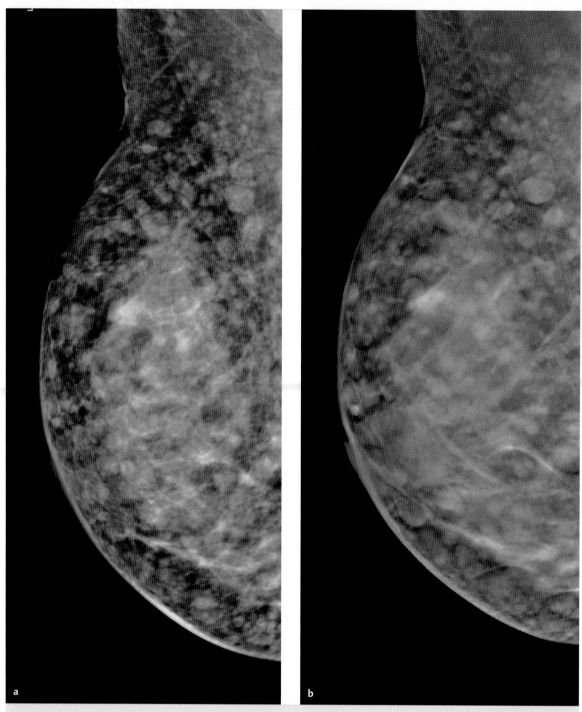

Fig. 5.39 Case 39. 40-year-old woman, first diagnosed 5 years earlier with multiple myeloma. Status post high-dose chemotherapy and stem-cell transplantation. Intramammary involvement 2 years earlier, treated by radiotherapy. Two-month history of bilateral, multiple, progressive palpable masses approximately 1 cm in size. **(a)** Digital mammogram of the right breast, MLO projection. **(b)** Single slice from 3D tomosynthesis data set of the right breast, MLO projection.

continued ▶

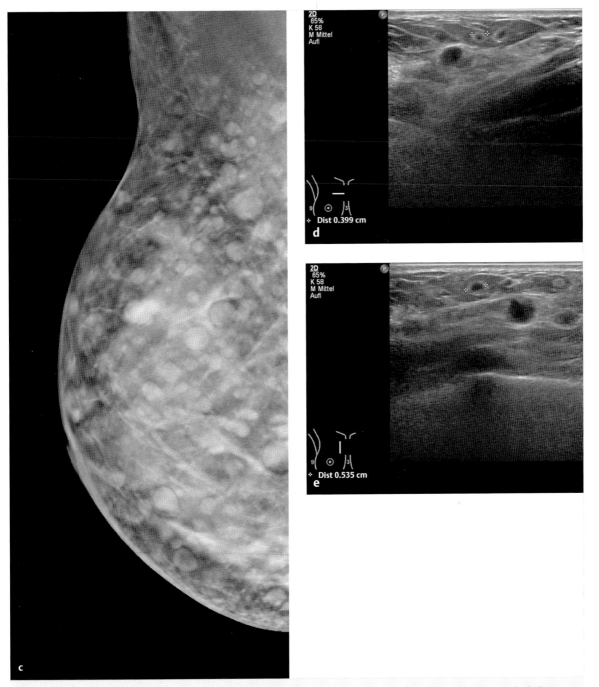

Fig. 5.39 (continued) Case 39. 40-year-old woman, first diagnosed 5 years earlier with multiple myeloma. Status post high-dose chemotherapy and stem-cell transplantation. Intramammary involvement 2 years earlier, treated by radiotherapy. Two-month history of bilateral, multiple, progressive palpable masses, approximately 1 cm in size. **(c)** Single slice from 3D tomosynthesis data set of the right breast, MLO projection. **(d)** Ultrasound scan of the masses in the upper inner quadrant of the right breast. **(e)** Ultrasound scan of the masses in the upper inner quadrant of the right breast.

continued ▶

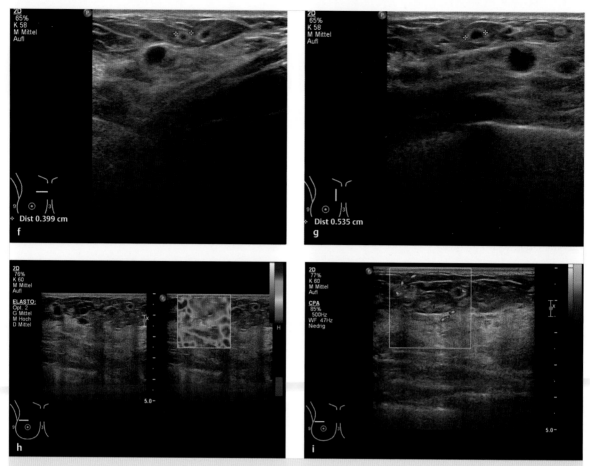

Fig. 5.39 (continued) Case 39. 40-year-old woman, first diagnosed 5 years earlier with multiple myeloma. Status post high-dose chemotherapy and stem-cell transplantation. Intramammary involvement 2 years earlier, treated by radiotherapy. Two-month history of bilateral, multiple, progressive palpable masses, approximately 1 cm in size. **(f)** Ultrasound scan of the masses in the upper inner quadrant of the right breast. **(g)** Ultrasound scan of the mass in the upper inner quadrant of the right breast. **(h)** Elastography of the masses in the upper outer quadrant of the right breast. **(i)** Power Doppler scan of the masses in the upper outer quadrant of the right breast.

5.2.40 Case 40

History

Woman 64 years of age. Family history of breast cancer, with a sister diagnosed at age 49 years. G2, P2, breastfed for 1 week and 7 months. Status post-biopsy with clip insertion in the left breast. Histology showed fibrocystic changes.

Mammography

Right breast: ACR 3. No masses or suspicious microcalcifications. Classified as BI-RADS 2 (**Fig. 5.40a, c**). Left breast: ACR 3. Central spiculated mass in the MLO view, with no definite correlate in the CC view. Biopsy clip in place. Classified as BI-RADS 4 (**Fig. 5.40b, d**).

DBT

MLO view of the left breast shows no evidence of a mass and no correlate for the spiculated mammographic lesion. The clip is also visible in tomosynthesis slices (**Fig. 5.40e, Video 5.20**).

Ultrasonography

Ultrasonography found no lesion correlating with the mammographic density.

Further Case History

The left breast was downgraded to BI-RADS 2, and the mammographic density was interpreted as a summation artifact. No evidence of breast cancer in later follow-ups.

Discussion

Tomosynthesis can reduce the need for further investigation by additional tests, core-needle biopsy, or short-term follow-ups. Several large studies have documented a reduction in recall rates.[3]

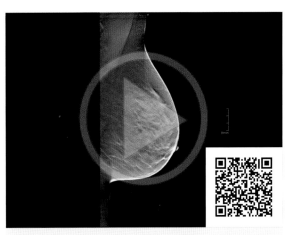

Video 5.20 Case 40. DBT data set of the left breast, MLO projection. No visible abnormalities, biopsy clip in place.

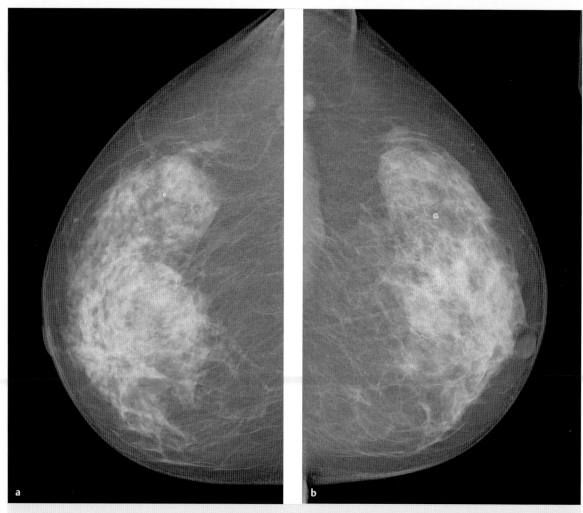

Fig. 5.40 Case 40. 64-year-old woman with family history of breast cancer. Status post-biopsy with clip insertion in the left breast. Histology showed fibrocystic changes. (a) Digital mammogram of the right breast, CC projection. (b) Digital mammogram of the left breast, CC projection.

continued ▶

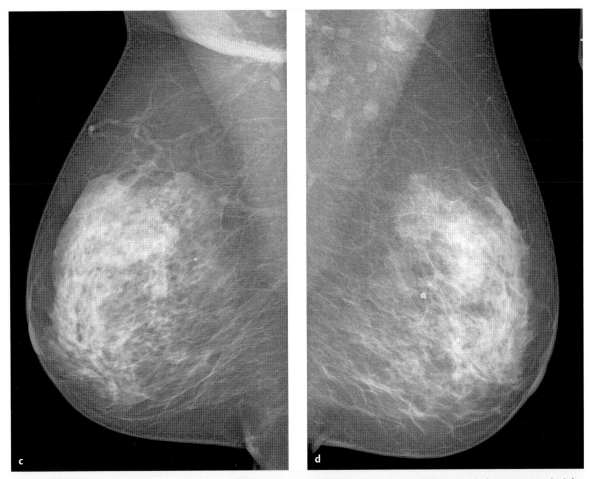

Fig. 5.40 (continued) Case 40. 64-year-old woman with family history of breast cancer. Status post-biopsy with clip insertion in the left breast. Histology showed fibrocystic changes. **(c)** Digital mammogram of the right breast, MLO projection. **(d)** Digital mammogram of the left breast, MLO projection.

continued ▶

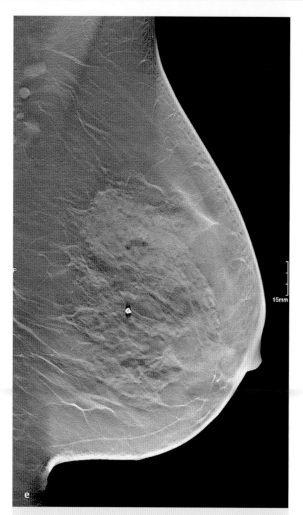

Fig. 5.40 (continued) Case 40. 64-year-old woman with family history of breast cancer. Status post-biopsy with clip insertion in the left breast. Histology showed fibrocystic changes. **(e)** Single slice from 3D tomosynthesis data set of the left breast, MLO projection. Clip is visible; no suspicious mass.

5.2.41 Case 41

History

Woman 60 years of age with a family history of breast cancer. Both breasts are normal in appearance, but both have palpable fibrocystic nodules. No nipple discharge or other abnormalities.

Mammography

Left breast: ACR 3. CC projection shows fibrocystic changes with no other abnormalities (**Fig. 5.41a**).

DBT

MLO view of the left breast shows a string-of-beads density of 12 × 4 mm, with well-defined margins 5 cm behind the nipple, suspicious for papillomatosis. The differential diagnosis includes duct ectasia and DCIS (**Fig. 5.41b, c**).

Ultrasonography

Elongated hypoechoic lesion at the 3 o'clock position, 11 × 5 mm, located 4 cm from the nipple. The nonperfused lesion correlates with the tomosynthesis finding. Suspicious for an intraductal mass. Differential diagnosis includes papilloma and DCIS (**Fig. 5.41d, e**).

Further Case History

Ultrasound-guided core-needle biopsy identified the lesion as papillomatosis.

Final Diagnosis

Papillomatosis, B3 lesion.

Discussion

In this case, tomosynthesis in the MLO projection was initially combined with mammography in the CC projection. An MLO mammogram was not obtained because DBT and ultrasonography both showed a suspicious lesion, which was biopsied under imaging guidance.

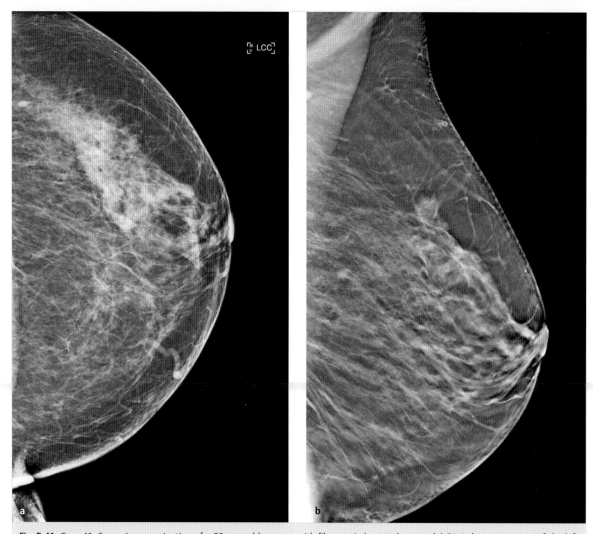

Fig. 5.41 Case 41. Screening examination of a 60-year-old woman with fibrocystic breast changes. **(a)** Digital mammogram of the left breast, CC projection. ACR density grade 3. **(b)** Single slice from 3D tomosynthesis data set of the left breast, MLO projection.

continued ▶

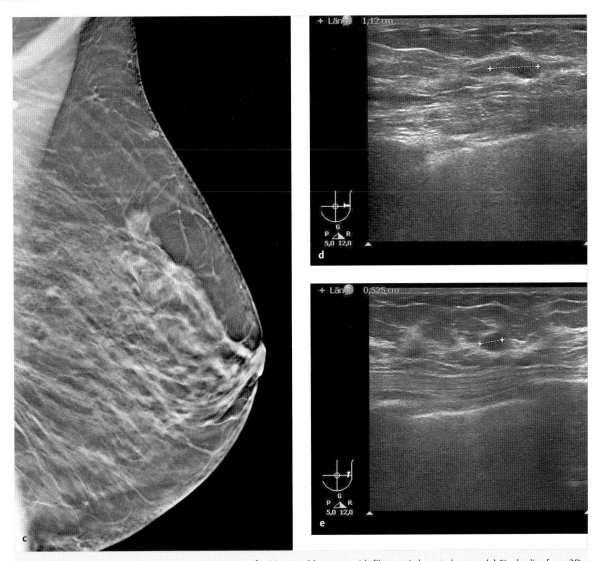

Fig. 5.41 (continued) Case 41. Screening examination of a 60-year-old woman with fibrocystic breast changes. **(c)** Single slice from 3D tomosynthesis data set of the left breast, MLO projection. **(d)** Ultrasound scan of the lesion at the 3 o'clock position in the left breast. **(e)** Ultrasound scan of the lesion at the 3 o'clock position in the left breast.

5.2.42 Case 42

History

Woman 40 years of age, no family history of breast cancer. Bloody right nipple discharge for several weeks. Palpation shows diffuse induration of the right breast compared with the left. The right nipple is flattened and blood-stained.

Mammography

Right breast: ACR 3. Standard mammogram in the MLO projection shows pleomorphic calcifications throughout the breast parenchyma. A lymph node of approximately 12 × 10 mm is visible in the axillary tail. Classified as BI-RADS 5 (**Fig. 5.42a**).

DBT

DBT of the right breast in the MLO projection. Some of the slices show pleomorphic, clustered calcifications (**Fig. 5.42b**), while other slices display the ductal arrangement of the calcifications, which is most apparent laterally (**Fig. 5.42c**) and caudally (**Fig. 5.42d**). Classified as BI-RADS 5.

Further Case History

The calcifications in the lower right breast were investigated by vacuum biopsy.

Final Diagnosis

High-grade DCIS with areas of comedonecrosis, B5 a lesion.

Discussion

Tomosynthesis, like mammography, can define the individual morphology of breast calcifications. Especially in case of numerous calcifications, tomosynthesis permits a more accurate assessment of their regional distribution pattern than mammography.

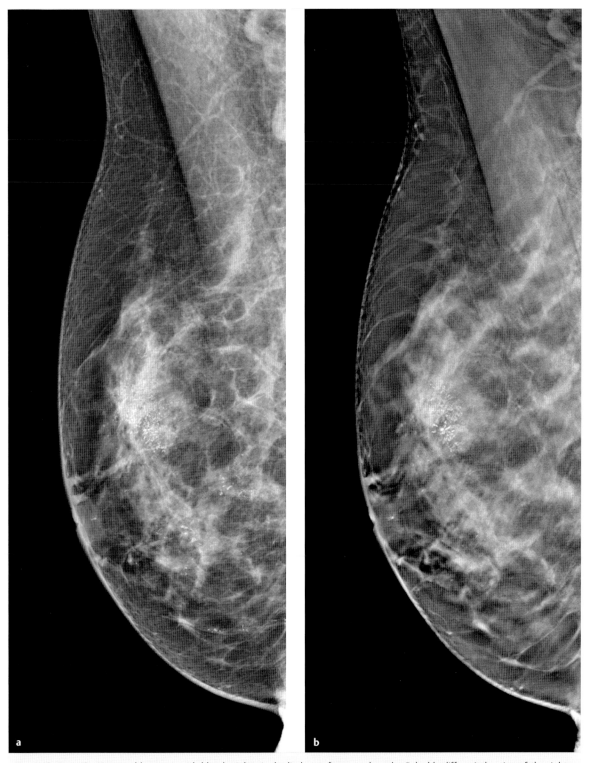

Fig. 5.42 Case 42. 40-year-old woman with bloody right nipple discharge for several weeks. Palpable diffuse induration of the right breast compared with the left. Right nipple is flattened and bloodstained. **(a)** Digital mammogram of the right breast, MLO projection. **(b)** Single slice from 3D tomosynthesis data set of the right breast, MLO projection.

continued ▶

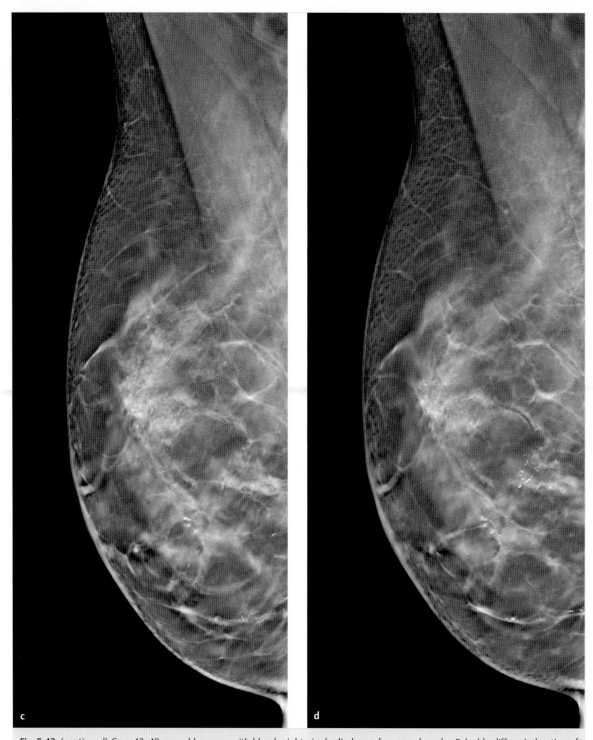

Fig. 5.42 (continued) Case 42. 40-year-old woman with bloody right nipple discharge for several weeks. Palpable diffuse induration of the right breast compared with the left. Right nipple is flattened and bloodstained. (c) Single slice from 3D tomosynthesis data set of the right breast, MLO projection. (d) Single slice from 3D tomosynthesis data set of the right breast, MLO projection.

5.2.43 Case 43

History

Woman 77 years of age with a family history of breast cancer (mother diagnosed after menopause). Patient is free of complaints but has palpable fibrocystic changes in both breasts. She has no visible breast abnormalities. The axillary lymph nodes are not enlarged.

Mammography

Right breast: ACR 3. Fine nodular pattern of fibrocystic changes. CC mammogram shows pleomorphic, predominantly rounded microcalcifications, 4 cm lateral to the nipple (**Fig. 5.43a**). A supplemental microfocus magnification view in a true-lateral projection also shows ductal calcifications covering an area of approximately 30 × 20 × 45 mm (**Fig. 5.43b**). Classified as BI-RADS 4b.

DBT

MLO view of the right breast shows predominantly retroareolar ductal calcifications. Solitary oval and rounded particles are also visualized in this area (**Fig. 5.43c, d**). Classified as BI-RADS 5.

Further Case History

The suspicious area was investigated by vacuum biopsy under stereotactic guidance.

Final Diagnosis

High-grade DCIS with comedonecrosis and associated microcalcifications. Final postoperative histology staged the tumor as pTis (45 mm).

Discussion

The calcifications shown by mammography and by the microfocus magnification view are also clearly defined by tomosynthesis. DBT is best for evaluating the regional distribution pattern of the pleomorphic calcifications. The detection of ductal calcifications by tomosynthesis strengthens the suspicion of DCIS, which was later confirmed histologically. It should be reemphasized, however, that individual DBT slices display only some of the microcalcifications. The entire cluster can be appreciated only by scrolling through the image stack or by using thick-slab maximum-intensity reconstructions.

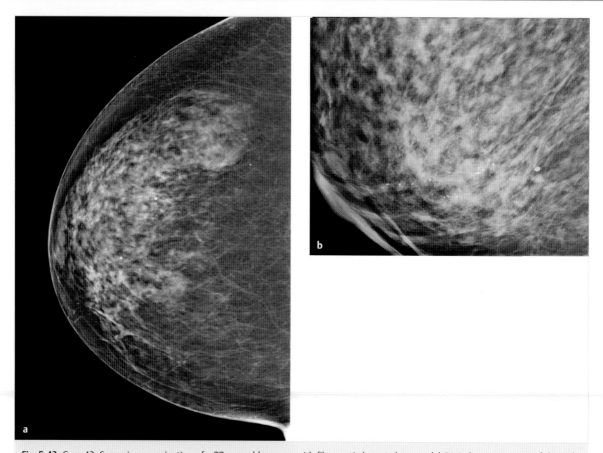

Fig. 5.43 Case 43. Screening examination of a 77-year-old woman with fibrocystic breast changes. **(a)** Digital mammogram of the right breast, CC projection. **(b)** Microfocus magnification view of the right breast, ML projection.

continued ▶

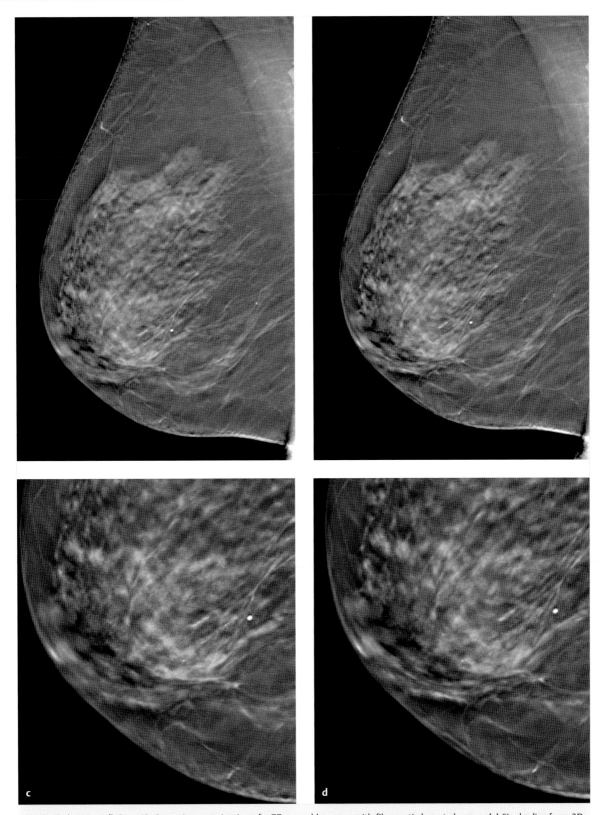

Fig. 5.43 (continued) Case 43. Screening examination of a 77-year-old woman with fibrocystic breast changes. **(c)** Single slice from 3D tomosynthesis data set of the right breast, MLO projection, with a magnified view of the suspicious area. **(d)** Single slice from 3D tomosynthesis data set of the right breast, MLO projection, with a magnified view of the suspicious area.

5.2.44 Case 44

History

Asymptomatic 50-year-old woman. G1, P1, breastfed for 8 weeks. She had her first period at age 15 years, a hysterectomy at age 38 years. Maternal history of breast cancer at age 44 years.

Mammography

Right breast: ACR 3. Lobulated mass with predominantly smooth margins at the 3 o'clock position. No suspicious masses or microcalcifications. Classified as BI-RADS 2 (**Fig. 5.44a, c**). Left breast: ACR 3. Spiculated lesion at the 6 o'clock position, with spicules radiating to the pectoralis muscle. No suspicious microcalcifications. Classified as BI-RADS 5 (**Fig. 5.44b, d**).

DBT

MLO view of the left breast shows a suspicious, 1.6-cm spiculated mass at the 4 o'clock position. Classified as BI-RADS 5 (**Fig. 5.44e, Video 5.21**). CC view of the right breast shows a lobulated mass with smooth margins that does not appear suspicious. Classified as BI-RADS 2 (**Fig. 5.44f, g**).

Ultrasonography

Left breast: Suspicious hypoechoic mass with ill-defined margins at the 4 o'clock position, measuring 1.4 × 1.5 × 1.2 cm (**Fig. 5.44h**). Right breast: The lobulated, smooth-bordered mass has been unchanged for 3 years and represents a fibroadenoma.

MRI

MRI Breast shows an enhancing lesion 12 cm behind the left nipple, with spicules radiating into the surrounding fat but no apparent invasion of the pectoralis muscle (**Fig. 5.44i**).

Further Case History

Core-needle biopsy confirmed a poorly differentiated invasive carcinoma (no special type) in the left breast.

Discussion

Tomosynthesis defines the smooth margins of the fibroadenoma and the radiating spicules of the carcinoma more clearly than mammography. However, neither can definitely confirm or exclude invasion of the pectoralis muscle. Supplemental MRI defines the tumor extent and can also exclude chest wall invasion.

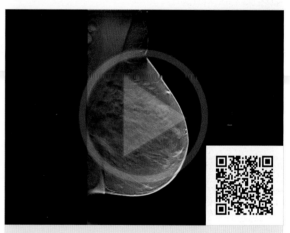

Video 5.21 Case 44. DBT data set of the left breast, MLO projection. A suspicious, 1.6-cm mass with radiating spicules is visible at the 4 o'clock position.

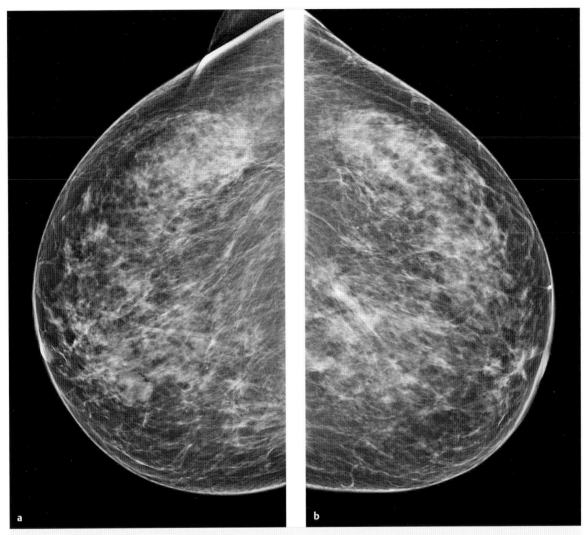

Fig. 5.44 Case 44. Screening examination of an asymptomatic 50-year-old woman. **(a)** Digital mammogram of the right breast, CC projection. **(b)** Digital mammogram of the left breast, CC projection.

continued ▶

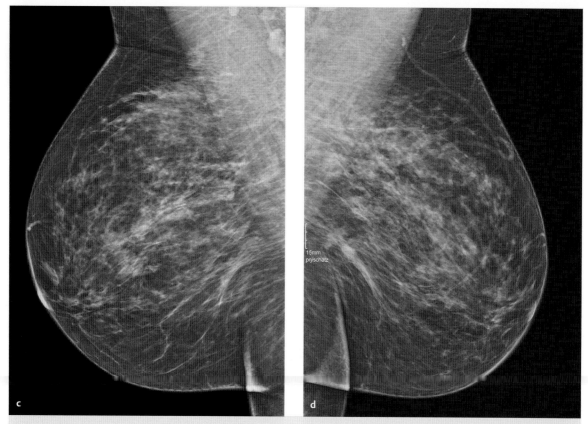

15mm
prj/schätz

Fig. 5.44 (continued) Case 44. Screening examination of an asymptomatic 50-year-old woman. **(c)** Digital mammogram of the right breast, MLO projection. **(d)** Digital mammogram of the left breast, MLO projection.

continued ▶

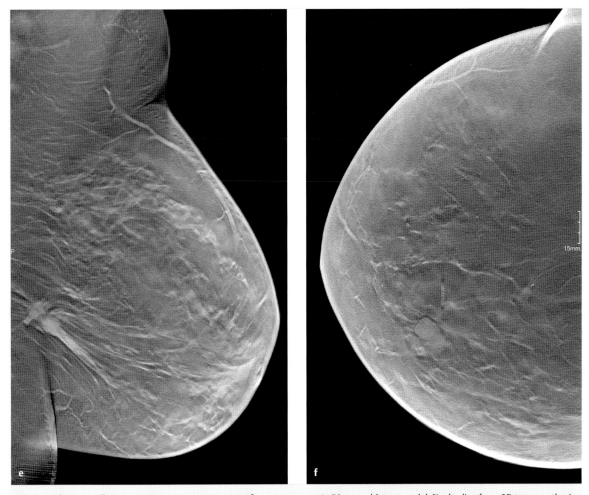

Fig. 5.44 (continued) Case 44. Screening examination of an asymptomatic 50-year-old woman. (e) Single slice from 3D tomosynthesis data set of the left breast, MLO projection. Carcinoma. (f) Single slice from 3D tomosynthesis data set of the right breast, CC projection. Fibroadenoma.

continued ▶

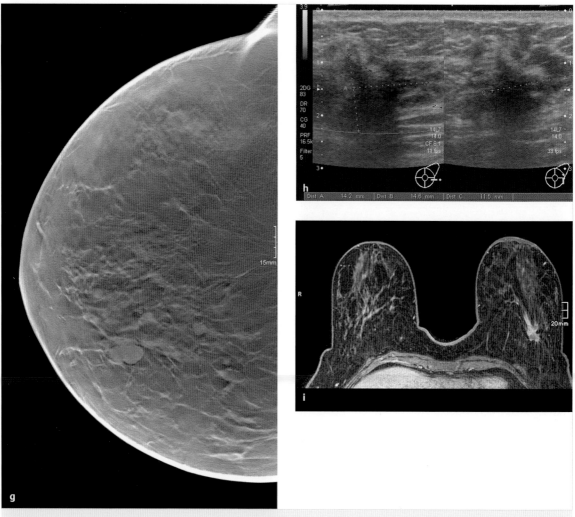

Fig. 5.44 (continued) Case 44. Screening examination of an asymptomatic 50-year-old woman. **(g)** Single slice from 3D tomosynthesis data set of the right breast, CC projection. Fibroadenoma. **(h)** Ultrasound scan of the lesion in the left breast. **(i)** High-resolution T 1-weighted fat-suppressed MRI, late phase after contrast administration.

5.2.45 Case 45

History

Woman 51 years of age with a family history of breast cancer (maternal aunt and grandmother). Nulliparous. She is free of complaints but has palpable fibrocystic nodularity. The breasts appear normal on inspection, with no enlarged axillary lymph nodes on either side.

Mammography

Right breast: ACR 3. Moderately coarse pattern of fibrocystic changes. CC view shows a questionable architectural distortion 6 cm lateral to the nipple. Classified as BI-RADS 4 (**Fig. 5.45a**).

DBT

DBT of the right breast in the CC and MLO projections. Both views clearly depict architectural distortion 6 cm lateral to the nipple. Classified as BI-RADS 5 (**Fig. 5.45b, c**).

Ultrasonography

A hypoechoic lesion measuring 20 × 5 × 15 mm, with a hyperechoic rim, is found at the 10 to 11 o'clock position in the right breast, 5 cm from the nipple. The lesion appears microlobulated, disrupts the Cooper's ligaments, and has an inhomogeneous acoustic shadow. Classified as BI-RADS 5 (**Fig. 5.45d, e**).

Further Case History

Ultrasound-guided core-needle biopsy identified the lesion histologically as tubular breast carcinoma (luminal A). Final postoperative histology staged the tumor at pT 1 c (18 mm) with associated low-grade intratumoral DCIS.

Discussion

The architectural distortion is difficult to evaluate on mammograms and is visible only in the CC projection, but it is clearly displayed in both the CC and MLO tomosynthesis views. When the patient is imaged by mammography alone, as in screening, DBT can be a valuable adjunct for detecting architectural distortion. When combined with ultrasonography in the present case, tomosynthesis did not add significant information since the ultrasonography findings alone provided an urgent indication for biopsy.

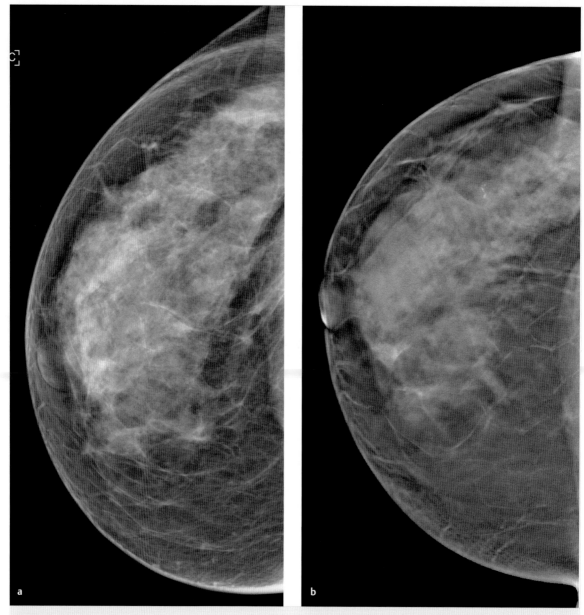

Fig. 5.45 Case 45. Screening examination of a 51-year-old woman with fibrocystic breast changes. **(a)** Digital mammogram of the right breast, CC projection. **(b)** Single slice from 3D tomosynthesis data set of the right breast, CC projection.

continued ▶

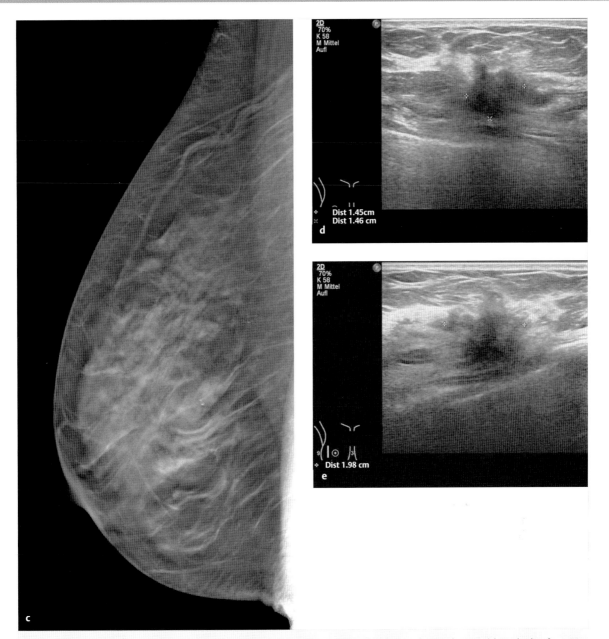

Fig. 5.45 (continued) Case 45. Screening examination of a 51-year-old woman with fibrocystic breast changes. **(c)** Single slice from 3D tomosynthesis data set of the right breast, MLO projection. **(d)** Ultrasound scan of the lesion (12.5-MHz probe). **(e)** Ultrasound scan of the lesion, second plane.

5.3 References

[1] Rafferty EA, Park JM, Philpotts LE et al. Assessing radiologist performance using combined digital mammography and breast tomosynthesis compared with digital mammography alone: results of a multicenter, multireader trial. Radiology 2013; 266: 104–113

[2] Bae MS, Moon WK, Chang JM et al. Breast cancer detected with screening US: reasons for nondetection at mammography. Radiology 2014; 270: 369–377

[3] Haas BM, Kalra V, Geisel J et al. Comparison of tomosynthesis plus digital mammography and digital mammography alone for breast cancer screening. Radiology 2013; 269: 697–700

Appendix

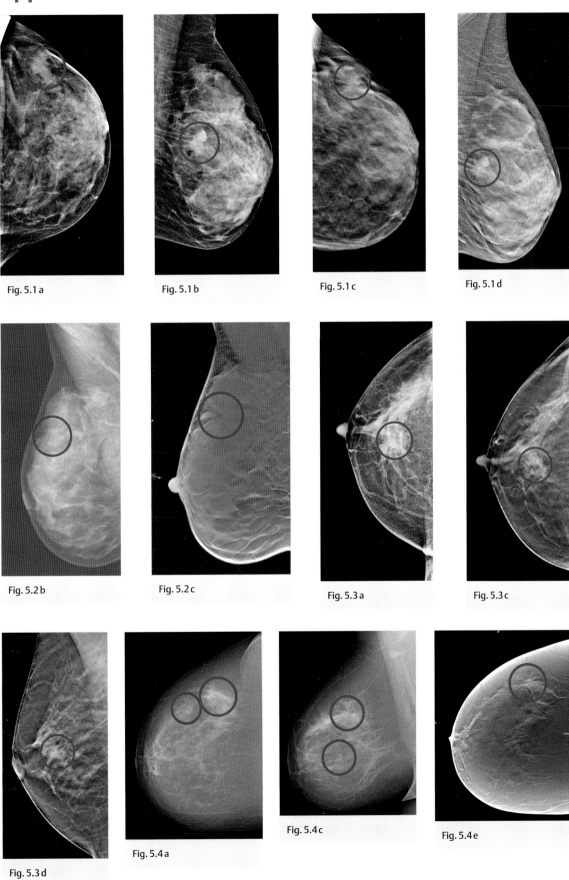

Fig. 5.1 a

Fig. 5.1 b

Fig. 5.1 c

Fig. 5.1 d

Fig. 5.2 b

Fig. 5.2 c

Fig. 5.3 a

Fig. 5.3 c

Fig. 5.3 d

Fig. 5.4 a

Fig. 5.4 c

Fig. 5.4 e

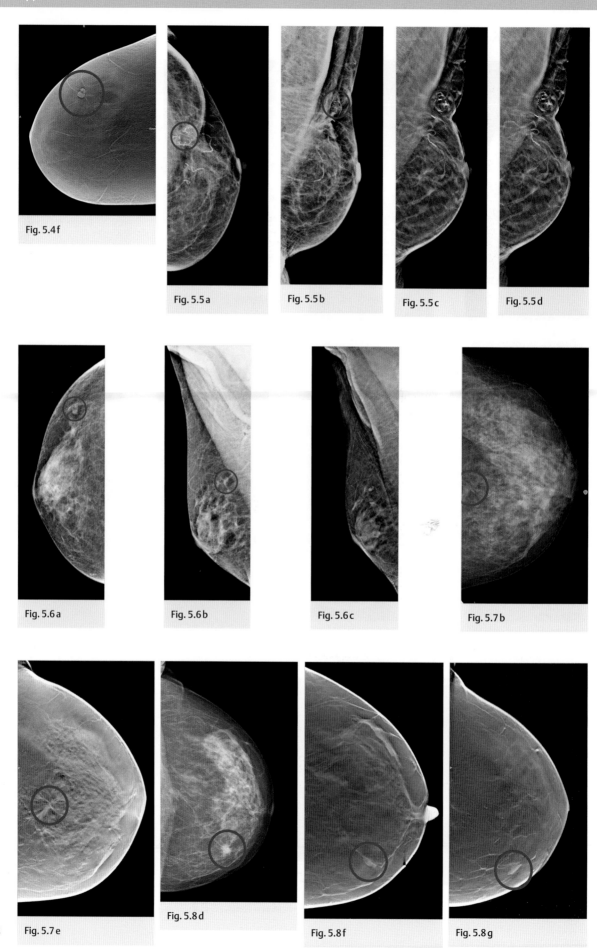

Fig. 5.4 f

Fig. 5.5 a

Fig. 5.5 b

Fig. 5.5 c

Fig. 5.5 d

Fig. 5.6 a

Fig. 5.6 b

Fig. 5.6 c

Fig. 5.7 b

Fig. 5.7 e

Fig. 5.8 d

Fig. 5.8 f

Fig. 5.8 g

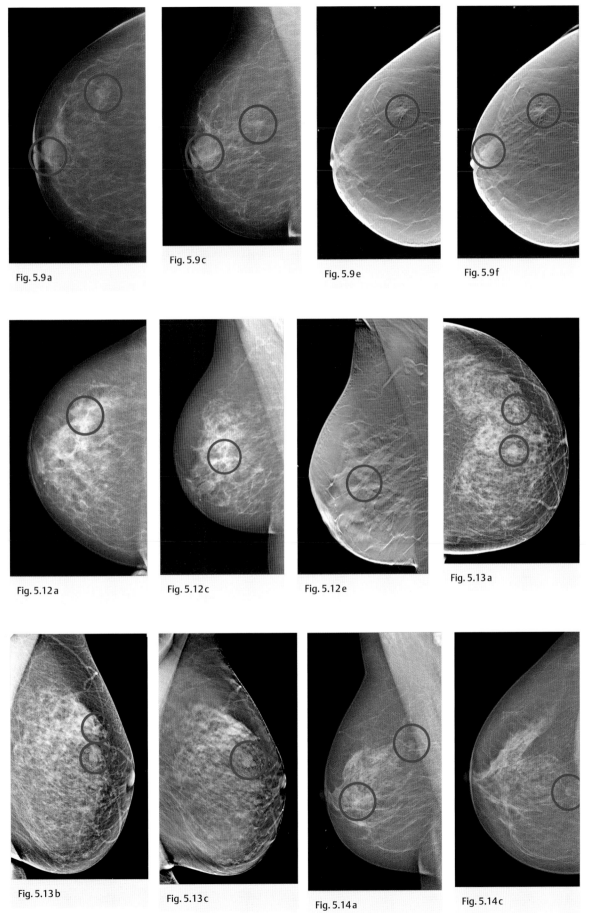

Fig. 5.9 a

Fig. 5.9 c

Fig. 5.9 e

Fig. 5.9 f

Fig. 5.12 a

Fig. 5.12 c

Fig. 5.12 e

Fig. 5.13 a

Fig. 5.13 b

Fig. 5.13 c

Fig. 5.14 a

Fig. 5.14 c

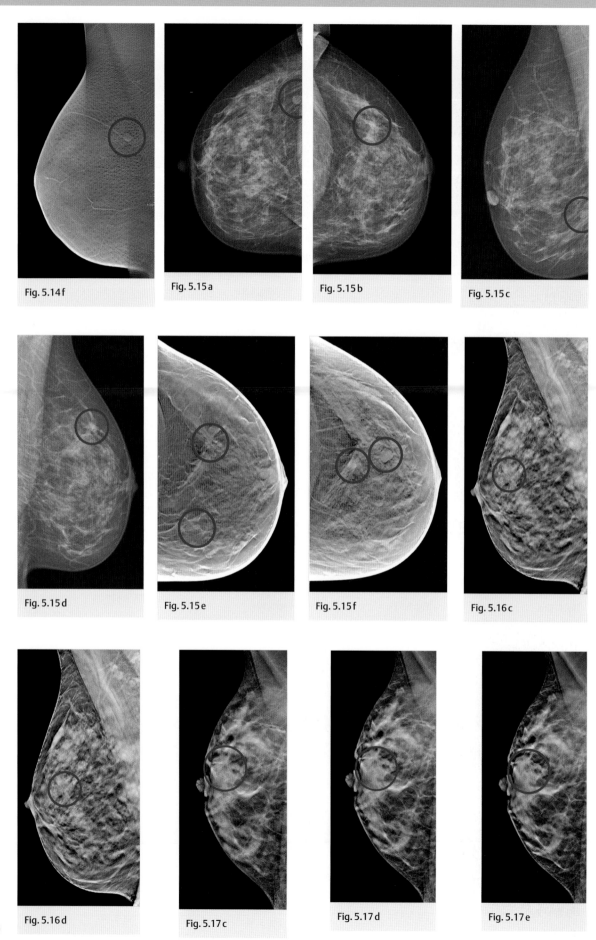

Fig. 5.14 f

Fig. 5.15 a

Fig. 5.15 b

Fig. 5.15 c

Fig. 5.15 d

Fig. 5.15 e

Fig. 5.15 f

Fig. 5.16 c

Fig. 5.16 d

Fig. 5.17 c

Fig. 5.17 d

Fig. 5.17 e

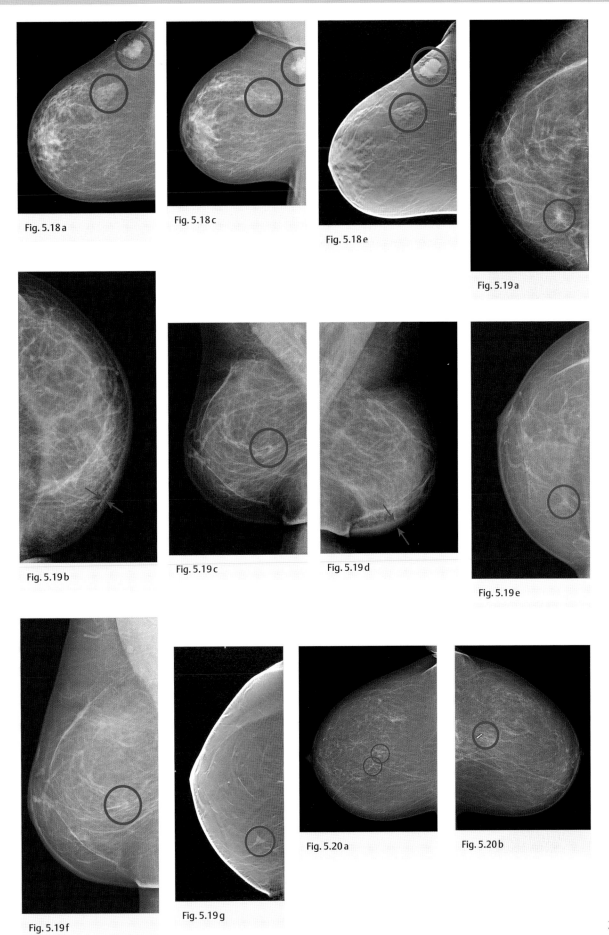

Fig. 5.18 a

Fig. 5.18 c

Fig. 5.18 e

Fig. 5.19 a

Fig. 5.19 b

Fig. 5.19 c

Fig. 5.19 d

Fig. 5.19 e

Fig. 5.19 f

Fig. 5.19 g

Fig. 5.20 a

Fig. 5.20 b

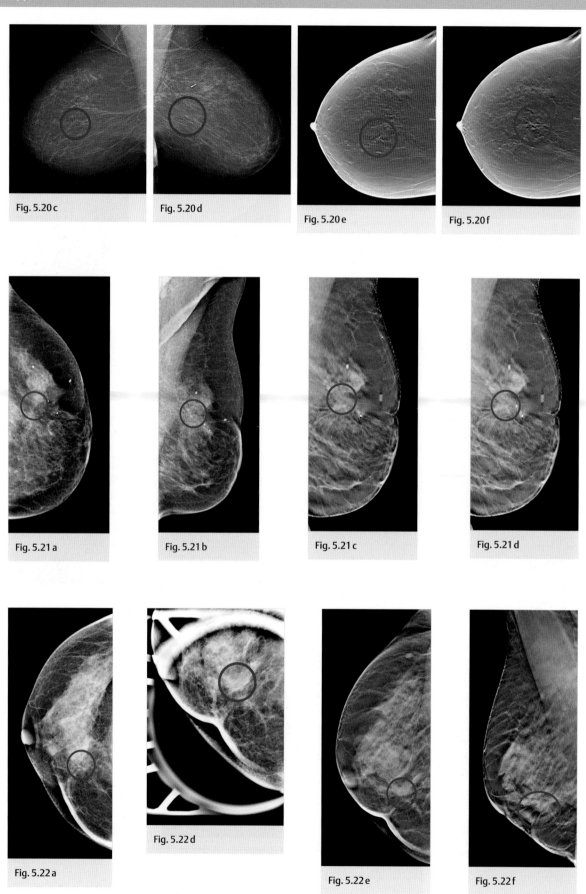

Fig. 5.20 c

Fig. 5.20 d

Fig. 5.20 e

Fig. 5.20 f

Fig. 5.21 a

Fig. 5.21 b

Fig. 5.21 c

Fig. 5.21 d

Fig. 5.22 a

Fig. 5.22 d

Fig. 5.22 e

Fig. 5.22 f

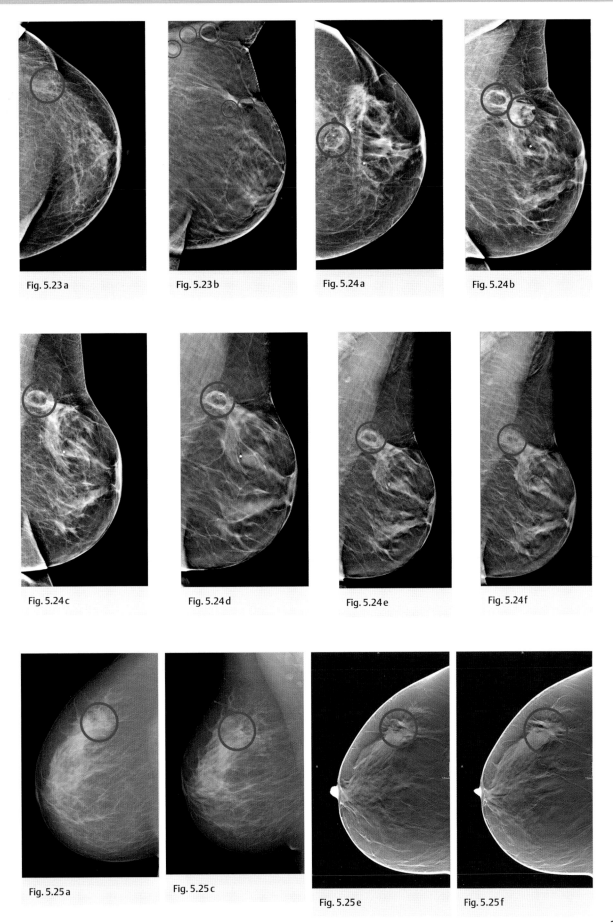

Fig. 5.23 a

Fig. 5.23 b

Fig. 5.24 a

Fig. 5.24 b

Fig. 5.24 c

Fig. 5.24 d

Fig. 5.24 e

Fig. 5.24 f

Fig. 5.25 a

Fig. 5.25 c

Fig. 5.25 e

Fig. 5.25 f

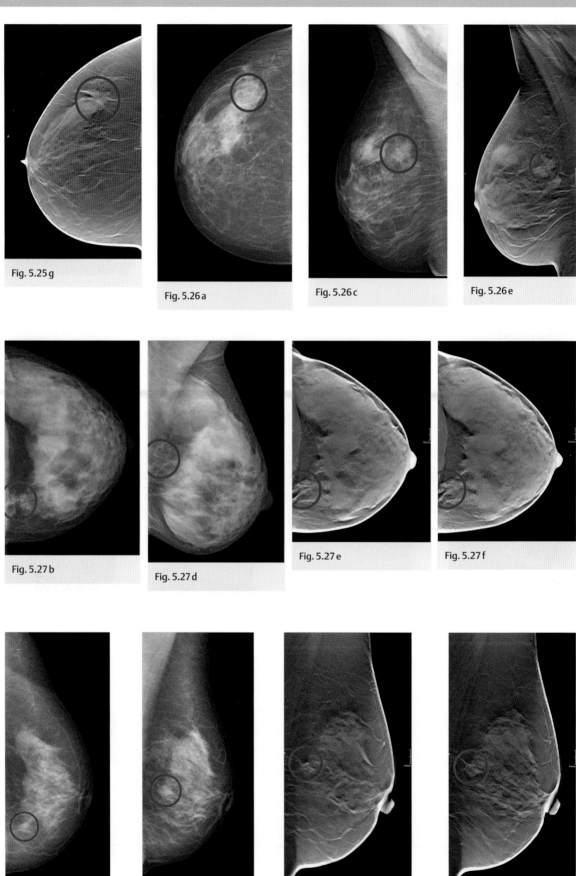

Fig. 5.25 g

Fig. 5.26 a

Fig. 5.26 c

Fig. 5.26 e

Fig. 5.27 b

Fig. 5.27 d

Fig. 5.27 e

Fig. 5.27 f

Fig. 5.28 b

Fig. 5.28 d

Fig. 5.28 e

Fig. 5.28 f

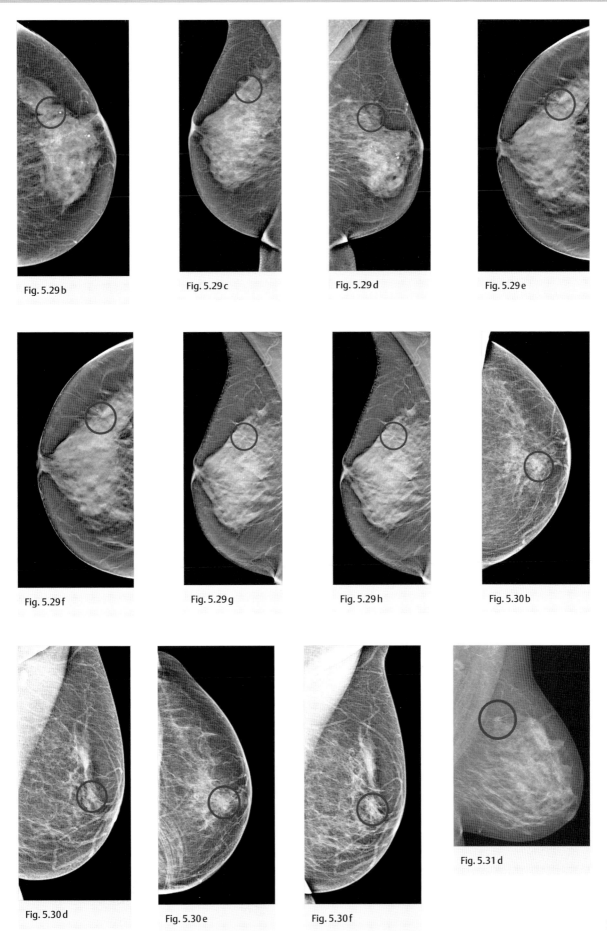

Fig. 5.29 b

Fig. 5.29 c

Fig. 5.29 d

Fig. 5.29 e

Fig. 5.29 f

Fig. 5.29 g

Fig. 5.29 h

Fig. 5.30 b

Fig. 5.30 d

Fig. 5.30 e

Fig. 5.30 f

Fig. 5.31 d

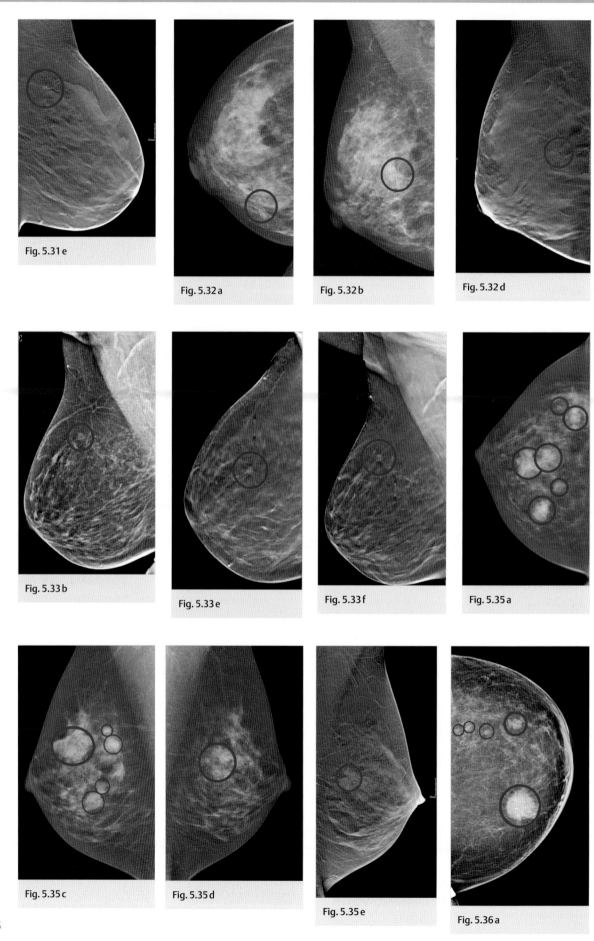

Fig. 5.31 e

Fig. 5.32 a

Fig. 5.32 b

Fig. 5.32 d

Fig. 5.33 b

Fig. 5.33 e

Fig. 5.33 f

Fig. 5.35 a

Fig. 5.35 c

Fig. 5.35 d

Fig. 5.35 e

Fig. 5.36 a

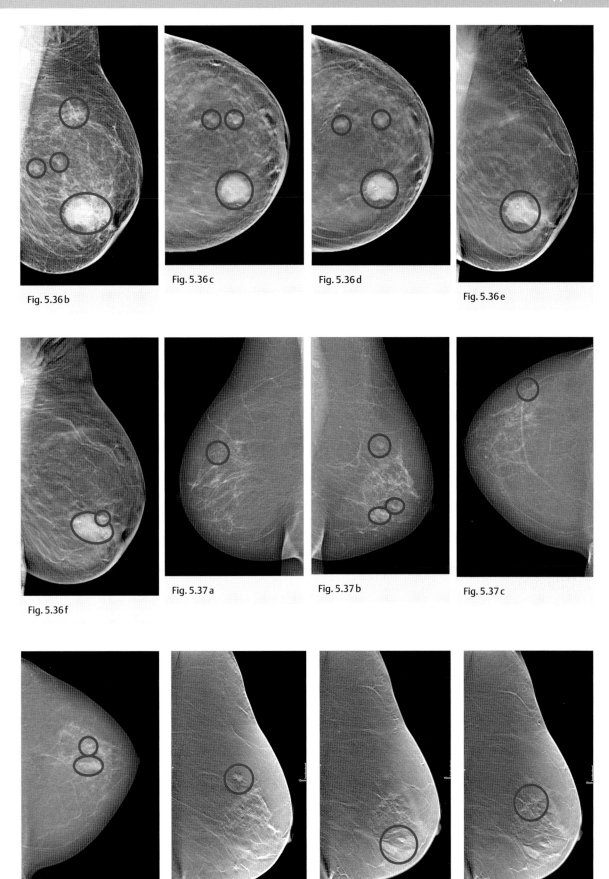

Fig. 5.36 b

Fig. 5.36 c

Fig. 5.36 d

Fig. 5.36 e

Fig. 5.36 f

Fig. 5.37 a

Fig. 5.37 b

Fig. 5.37 c

Fig. 5.37 d

Fig. 5.37 e

Fig. 5.37 f

Fig. 5.37 g

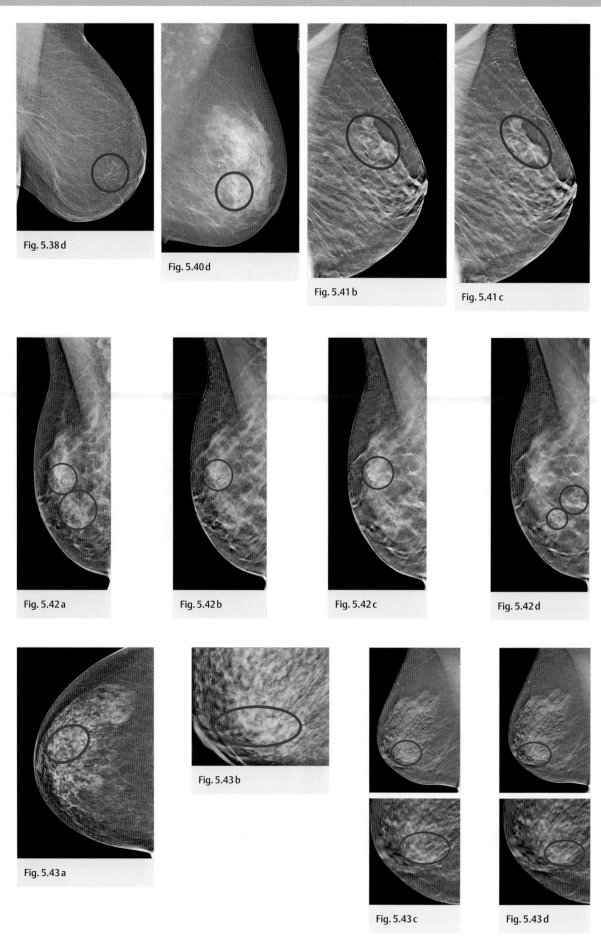

Fig. 5.38 d

Fig. 5.40 d

Fig. 5.41 b

Fig. 5.41 c

Fig. 5.42 a

Fig. 5.42 b

Fig. 5.42 c

Fig. 5.42 d

Fig. 5.43 a

Fig. 5.43 b

Fig. 5.43 c

Fig. 5.43 d

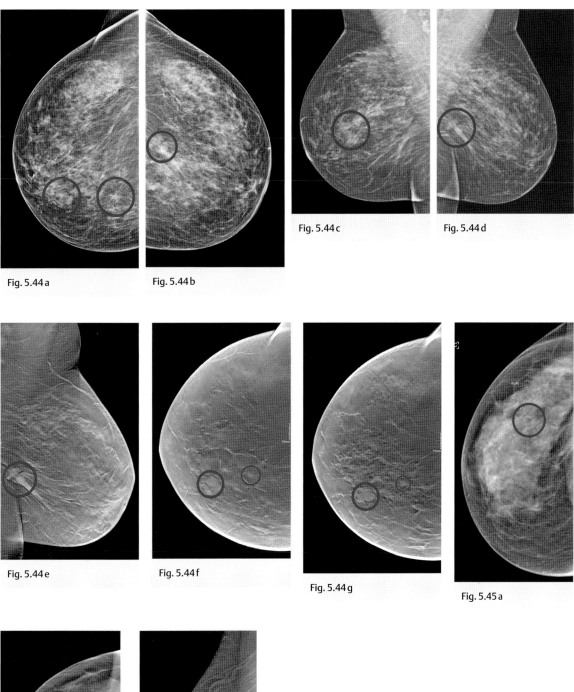

Fig. 5.44 a

Fig. 5.44 b

Fig. 5.44 c

Fig. 5.44 d

Fig. 5.44 e

Fig. 5.44 f

Fig. 5.44 g

Fig. 5.45 a

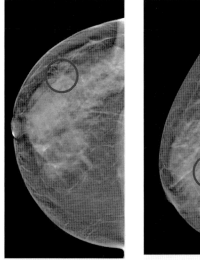

Fig. 5.45 b

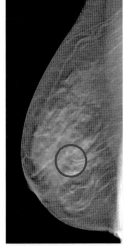

Fig. 5.45 c

Index

Page numbers in *italics* refer to illustrations